DIVINE NUTRITION: BIBLICAL DIETS FOR MODERN HEALTH CHALLENGES

NORMAN CALDWELL

Copyright © [2024] by NORMAN CALDWELL

All rights reserved.

No portion of this book may be reproduced in any form without written permission from the publisher or author, except as permitted by U.S. copyright law.

Contents

1. Introduction — 1
2. Part 1: Understanding Biblical Nutrition — 6
3. CHAPTER 1. The Biblical Basis for Healthy Eating — 7
4. CHAPTER 2. Clean and Unclean Foods — 13
5. Chapter 3: Feasting and Fasting in the Bible — 20
6. Part 2: Biblical Diet for Diabetes — 27
7. Chapter 4. Diabetes in Biblical Context — 28
8. Chapter 5: Foods to Include — 36
9. Chapter 6: Foods to Avoid — 44
10. Part 3: Biblical Diet for High Blood Pressure — 51
11. Chapter 7: High Blood Pressure in Biblical Context — 52
12. Chapter 8: Foods to Include — 61
13. Chapter 9: Foods to Avoid — 75
14. Part 4: Biblical Diet for Cholesterol — 85

15.	Chapter 10: Cholesterol in Biblical Context	86
16.	Chapter 11: Foods to Include	94
17.	Chapter 12: Foods to Avoid	104
18.	Part 5: Biblical Diet for Mental Health	113
19.	Chapter 13: Mental Health in Biblical Context	114
20.	Chapter 14: Foods to Include	123
21.	Chapter 15: Foods to Avoid	133
22.	Part 6: Practical Application	142
23.	Chapter 16: Meal Planning and Preparation	143
24.	Chapter 17: Incorporating Biblical Principles in Daily Life	152
25.	Chapter 18: Modern Recipes with Biblical Ingredients	163
26.	Chapter 19: Testimonials and Case Studies	174
27.	Chapter 20: Conclusion and Call to Action	183
28.	References for "Divine Nutrition: Biblical Principles for Modern Health"	192

Introduction

Overview of the Relevance of Biblical Dietary Principles in Modern Health

The Bible, a timeless and divine guide, offers profound wisdom on various aspects of life, including diet and nutrition. Its teachings are not only spiritually enriching but also hold significant relevance for modern health. By examining the dietary principles outlined in the Bible, we can uncover valuable insights that align with contemporary scientific understanding and address current health challenges.

Biblical dietary principles emphasize moderation, balance, and the consumption of whole, natural foods. These principles are echoed in modern nutritional science, which advocates for a balanced diet rich in fruits, vegetables, whole grains, lean proteins, and healthy fats. For instance, the Bible's emphasis on plant-based foods can be seen in Genesis 1:29: "And God said, Behold, I have given you every herb bearing seed, which is upon the face of all the earth, and every tree, in the which is the fruit of a tree yielding seed; to you it shall be for meat." This ancient directive highlights the importance of plant-based nutrition, a concept that is increasingly supported by modern research as beneficial for preventing and managing chronic diseases.

Explanation of the Connection Between Diet, Health, and Spirituality

The connection between diet, health, and spirituality is deeply intertwined in biblical teachings. The Bible often links physical health to spiritual well-being, suggesting that taking care of our bodies is a form of honoring God. 1 Corinthians 6:19-20 reminds us, "Do you not know that your bodies are temples of the Holy Spirit, who is in you, whom you have received from God? You are not your own; you were bought at a price. Therefore honor God with your bodies."

This passage underscores the spiritual responsibility of maintaining our health. By choosing nutritious foods and maintaining a healthy lifestyle, we are not only caring for our physical bodies but also nurturing our spiritual well-being. This holistic approach aligns with modern health perspectives that recognize the mind-body-spirit connection. Studies have shown that a healthy diet can improve mental health, reduce stress, and enhance overall quality of life, reinforcing the biblical view that our physical and spiritual health are interconnected.

Brief Introduction to Diabetes, High Blood Pressure, Cholesterol, and Mental Health

Modern health challenges such as diabetes, high blood pressure, cholesterol, and mental health issues are prevalent and often interrelated. These conditions are significantly influenced by diet and lifestyle, making the exploration of biblical dietary principles highly relevant.

1. **Diabetes**: Diabetes is a chronic condition characterized by elevated blood sugar levels. It can lead to serious complications if not managed properly. A diet high in processed sugars and refined carbohydrates can contribute to the development of diabetes. Biblical teachings on moderation and the consumption of natural, unprocessed foods can guide us in making healthier dietary choices. For example, Proverbs 25:16 warns, "Have you found honey? Eat only as much as you need, Lest you be filled with it and vomit." This advice on moderation is crucial for managing blood sugar levels.

2. **High Blood Pressure**: Hypertension, or high blood pressure, is a major risk factor for heart disease and stroke. A diet high in sodium and low in essential nutrients can contribute to hypertension. The Bible's emphasis on fruits, vegetables, and whole foods aligns with dietary recommendations for lowering blood pressure. Daniel 1:12 provides an example of a plant-based diet: "Please test your servants for ten days, and let them give us vegetables to eat and water to drink." This diet, rich in potassium and low in sodium, is beneficial for maintaining healthy blood pressure levels.

3. **Cholesterol**: Elevated cholesterol levels can lead to heart disease. A diet high in saturated fats and trans fats can increase cholesterol levels. The Bible's guidance on clean and unclean foods, as outlined in Leviticus 11, encourages the consumption of healthier, leaner meats and avoiding foods that are detrimental to health. Additionally, Ezekiel 47:12 highlights the healing properties of natural foods: "Their fruit will serve

for food and their leaves for healing." Incorporating fruits and vegetables into the diet can help manage cholesterol levels.

4. **Mental Health**: Mental health issues, including anxiety and depression, are increasingly common. Diet plays a crucial role in mental well-being. Foods rich in omega-3 fatty acids, antioxidants, and other nutrients can support brain health. The Bible recognizes the importance of mental well-being, as seen in 1 Kings 19:5-8, where Elijah is provided with food for strength during a time of despair. This story illustrates the restorative power of nourishment for both physical and mental health.

How to Use This Book for Practical, Spiritual, and Health Benefits

This book is designed to provide a comprehensive guide to integrating biblical dietary principles with modern nutritional science to address common health issues. By following the guidance in this book, readers can achieve practical, spiritual, and health benefits in the following ways:

1. **Practical Benefits**: The book offers practical advice on meal planning, food preparation, and dietary choices based on biblical teachings. By incorporating these principles into daily life, readers can improve their overall health and well-being. For example, the emphasis on whole, natural foods can help readers make healthier choices in their diet, leading to better management of diabetes, high blood pressure, cholesterol, and mental health.

2. **Spiritual Benefits**: By aligning dietary choices with biblical teachings, readers can deepen their spiritual connection and sense of purpose. Understanding that caring for one's body is a form of honoring God can provide motivation and fulfillment. The spiritual discipline of fasting, for instance, can be practiced not only for physical benefits but also as a way to draw closer to God.

3. **Health Benefits**: The book provides evidence-based insights into how biblical dietary principles can improve health outcomes. For example, the consumption of plant-based foods, as recommended in the Bible, is supported by modern research as beneficial for managing chronic diseases. By following these dietary guidelines, readers can experience improved physical health, reduced risk of chronic diseases, and enhanced mental well-being.

Conclusion

The intersection of biblical teachings and modern nutritional science offers a unique and innovative approach to addressing contemporary health challenges. By understanding and applying biblical dietary principles, we can achieve holistic health that encompasses physical, spiritual, and mental well-being. This book serves as a guide to integrating these timeless principles into our daily lives, providing practical, spiritual, and health benefits that are relevant for today's world.

PART 1: UNDERSTANDING BIBLICAL NUTRITION

CHAPTER 1. THE BIBLICAL BASIS FOR HEALTHY EATING

Genesis 1:29 – "And God said, Behold, I have given you every herb bearing seed, which is upon the face of all the earth, and every tree, in the which is the fruit of a tree yielding seed; to you it shall be for meat."

This verse, nestled within the creation narrative, sets the stage for understanding God's original design for human nutrition. It highlights a diet composed primarily of plant-based foods, an approach that resonates with contemporary nutritional science and health trends.

Overview of Plant-Based Diets in the Bible

The concept of a plant-based diet is deeply embedded in biblical text. From the Garden of Eden to the dietary laws of the Israelites, the Bible consistently underscores the benefits of consuming foods that are whole, natural, and unprocessed. Genesis 1:29 introduces us to God's initial provision for humanity: a diet rich in herbs, seeds, and fruits. This directive reflects a harmonious relationship between humans and the earth, emphasizing sustainability and health.

1. **The Garden of Eden**:

- In Genesis 2:8-9, we read about the Garden of Eden, where God planted every tree that is pleasant to the sight and good for food. The text specifies that "the tree of life was also in the midst of the garden, and the tree of the knowledge of good and evil." This idyllic setting underscores the abundance and variety of plant-based foods available to Adam and Eve. The fruit of these trees was not only for sustenance but also symbolized spiritual nourishment and life.

1. **The Diet of Daniel and His Friends**:

- In Daniel 1:12, we see a compelling example of a plant-based diet. Daniel and his friends chose to eat vegetables and drink water rather than partake in the royal food and wine, which were likely rich and possibly unclean by Jewish dietary laws. This decision led to their enhanced health and appearance compared to those who consumed the king's food. The story highlights the benefits of a simple, plant-based diet, which was instrumental in maintaining their health and faithfulness to God's commandments.

1. **Levitical Dietary Laws**:

- Leviticus 11 and Deuteronomy 14 outline the laws of clean and unclean animals. These guidelines were given to the Israelites to promote health and distinguish them as a holy people. The focus on clean animals, while prohibiting others, suggests a practical approach to food safety and health. These laws, though specific to the Israelites, also reflect broader principles of hygiene and dietary wisdom that are applicable today.

1. **The Promised Land's Abundance**:

o   Deuteronomy 8:7-8 describes the land flowing with milk and honey, abundant in wheat, barley, vines, fig trees, pomegranates, olive oil, and honey. This description emphasizes the nutritional richness and diversity of the foods available in the Promised Land, aligning with a diet that is both balanced and abundant in essential nutrients.

Modern Relevance: Emphasis on Plant-Based Diets and Their Benefits

In the contemporary world, the emphasis on plant-based diets is gaining momentum, supported by extensive research and growing health trends. The biblical endorsement of such diets is particularly relevant today, offering a timeless guide to improving health and well-being.

1. **Scientific Evidence Supporting Plant-Based Diets**:

o   **Cardiovascular Health**: Numerous studies have shown that plant-based diets are associated with a reduced risk of heart disease. The Adventist Health Study, for instance, found that individuals who followed a vegetarian or vegan diet had lower rates of heart disease compared to those who consumed meat. This aligns with the biblical principle of consuming a diet rich in fruits, vegetables, and whole grains.

o   **Diabetes Prevention and Management**: Research published in the American Journal of Clinical Nutrition indicates that plant-based diets can improve insulin sensitivity and reduce the risk of type 2 diabetes. The dietary patterns described in Genesis 1:29 and Daniel's diet highlight the benefits of a diet low in refined sugars and high in fiber and phytochemicals.

- **Cancer Risk Reduction**: The World Health Organization's International Agency for Research on Cancer (IARC) has classified processed meats as carcinogenic to humans. Conversely, plant-based diets, rich in antioxidants, fiber, and phytochemicals, have been shown to lower the risk of various cancers. This is consistent with the biblical emphasis on consuming a variety of fruits, vegetables, and whole grains.

1. **Nutritional Benefits of a Plant-Based Diet**:

- **Rich in Nutrients**: Plant-based diets are high in essential vitamins, minerals, and antioxidants. Foods like leafy greens, berries, nuts, and seeds provide a wealth of nutrients that support overall health. For example, leafy greens are rich in magnesium, potassium, and folate, which are crucial for cardiovascular health and cellular function.
- **Fiber-Rich**: High fiber intake is associated with numerous health benefits, including improved digestion, weight management, and lower cholesterol levels. The biblical diet, rich in fruits, vegetables, and whole grains, naturally provides ample fiber. Fiber helps regulate blood sugar levels and supports a healthy gut microbiome, enhancing immune function and reducing inflammation.

1. **Environmental and Ethical Considerations**:

- The Bible's emphasis on stewardship of the earth aligns with contemporary concerns about sustainability and environmental conservation. A plant-based diet is not only beneficial for individual health but also for the planet. According to the United Nations Food and Agriculture Organization (FAO), livestock production is a significant contributor to greenhouse gas emissions, deforestation, and water pollution. Embracing a plant-based diet can reduce our ecological footprint and promote sustainable living.

1. **Spiritual Implications**:

    o   The biblical call to eat a diet of fruits, vegetables, and grains is more than a health directive; it is a spiritual journey. In Deuteronomy 8:3, we read, "Man shall not live by bread alone, but by every word that proceeds from the mouth of the Lord." This verse reminds us that our spiritual nourishment is as crucial as our physical sustenance. A plant-based diet, rich in natural foods, can enhance our spiritual vitality, fostering a deeper connection with God and His creation.

Practical Application of Biblical Nutrition

Understanding the biblical basis for healthy eating and its modern relevance empowers us to make informed dietary choices that honor God and promote health. Here are some practical steps to incorporate biblical principles into our daily lives:

1. **Incorporate More Plant-Based Foods**:

    o   Aim to fill half your plate with fruits and vegetables at every meal. Choose a variety of colors and types to ensure a broad spectrum of nutrients. For example, start your day with a smoothie bowl topped with berries, spinach, and chia seeds.

1. **Adopt a Whole Foods Approach**:

    o   Focus on whole, unprocessed foods. Replace refined grains with whole grains like quinoa, brown rice, and oats. Choose legumes, nuts, and seeds as protein sources, and incorporate a variety of fruits and vegetables into your meals.

1. **Practice Moderation and Mindfulness**:

- Embrace the biblical principle of moderation. Proverbs 25:16 advises, "Have you found honey? Eat only as much as you need, lest you be filled with it and vomit." Practice mindful eating, savoring each bite and listening to your body's hunger and fullness cues.

1. **Engage in Fasting and Prayer**:

- Incorporate fasting into your spiritual routine, following the example of Daniel and Jesus. Fasting can enhance mental clarity, improve metabolic health, and deepen your spiritual connection. Use fasting as a time for prayer, reflection, and seeking God's guidance.

1. **Educate and Share**:

- Share your knowledge and experiences with others. Host a Bible study or cooking class focused on biblical nutrition. Encourage your community to explore plant-based diets and the health benefits they offer, fostering a supportive environment for healthy living.

The biblical basis for healthy eating, as outlined in Genesis 1:29 and other scriptures, provides a robust framework for understanding the benefits of a plant-based diet. This approach is not only supported by modern science but also aligns with spiritual principles that enhance our well-being. By embracing these biblical dietary guidelines, we can experience improved health, deepen our spiritual journey, and contribute to the well-being of our planet. Let us embark on this journey with faith, gratitude, and a commitment to living in harmony with God's creation.

CHAPTER 2. CLEAN AND UNCLEAN FOODS

Leviticus 11 – Guidelines on Clean and Unclean Foods

Leviticus 11 provides a detailed account of the dietary laws given to the Israelites, specifying which animals are considered clean and suitable for consumption and which are unclean and should be avoided. These laws were part of the larger covenantal relationship between God and Israel, intended to set them apart as a holy people. The chapter outlines the criteria for determining the cleanliness of land animals, sea creatures, birds, and insects.

Land Animals:

- Clean animals are those that both chew the cud and have a split hoof completely divided. Examples include cattle, sheep, and goats. (Leviticus 11:3)
- Unclean animals include those that do not meet both criteria, such as camels, rabbits, and pigs. (Leviticus 11:4-7)

Sea Creatures:

- Clean sea creatures are those that have fins and scales. Examples include fish like salmon and trout. (Leviticus 11:9)
- Unclean sea creatures include those without fins and scales, such as shellfish, crabs, and lobsters. (Leviticus 11:10-12)

Birds:

- The text lists specific birds that are considered unclean, including eagles, vultures, and owls. Clean birds are not explicitly listed, but by exclusion, birds such as chickens and turkeys are considered clean. (Leviticus 11:13-19)

Insects:

- Clean insects include those that have jointed legs for hopping, such as locusts, crickets, and grasshoppers. Other insects are considered unclean. (Leviticus 11:20-23)

These dietary laws were not arbitrary; they had practical implications for health and hygiene. By adhering to these guidelines, the Israelites could avoid many health risks associated with consuming certain animals.

Explanation of Clean Foods and Their Health Benefits

The distinction between clean and unclean foods in Leviticus 11 has significant health implications. Modern science supports many of these ancient guidelines, demonstrating the wisdom inherent in these dietary laws.

Clean Land Animals:

- **Nutritional Benefits**: Animals that chew the cud and have split hooves, such as cattle and sheep, typically have a diet that includes grasses and other vegetation, leading to leaner meat with a healthier fat profile. This meat is often rich in omega-3 fatty acids, which are beneficial for heart health.

- **Disease Prevention**: Clean animals are generally less prone to diseases that can be transmitted to humans. For example, pigs, which are considered unclean, are known carriers of parasites and diseases like trichinosis, which can be transmitted to humans through undercooked pork.

Clean Sea Creatures:

- **Nutritional Benefits**: Fish with fins and scales, such as salmon and mackerel, are excellent sources of protein, omega-3 fatty acids, and essential vitamins and minerals. These nutrients support cardiovascular health, brain function, and overall well-being.
- **Reduced Contamination Risk**: Fish without scales, such as catfish and shellfish, are more likely to absorb contaminants from their environment, including heavy metals and toxins. Consuming fish with fins and scales reduces the risk of exposure to these harmful substances.

Clean Birds:

- **Nutritional Benefits**: Poultry such as chicken and turkey provides high-quality protein, essential amino acids, and important nutrients like B vitamins and selenium. These birds are also relatively low in fat, particularly when the skin is removed.
- **Lower Disease Risk**: Birds listed as unclean in Leviticus 11, such as scavengers and birds of prey, are more likely to carry diseases and parasites due to their diet and lifestyle. Clean birds, which are typically domesticated and raised for consumption, pose fewer health risks.

Clean Insects:

- **Nutritional Benefits**: Edible insects like locusts and grasshoppers are high in protein, healthy fats, and essential nutrients like iron and zinc. In many cultures, insects are a sustainable and nutritious food source.

- **Sustainable Protein Source**: Insects require fewer resources to raise compared to traditional livestock, making them an environmentally friendly option for meeting protein needs.

Modern Relevance: Understanding Food Safety and Hygiene

The dietary laws in Leviticus 11 reflect a profound understanding of food safety and hygiene, principles that remain highly relevant in modern times. By examining these guidelines through the lens of contemporary science, we can appreciate their enduring value and applicability.

Food Safety:

- **Prevention of Foodborne Illnesses**: Many of the animals deemed unclean in Leviticus 11 are known carriers of pathogens that can cause foodborne illnesses. For instance, shellfish can harbor harmful bacteria and viruses, while pork can carry parasites like Trichinella spiralis. Avoiding these foods reduces the risk of consuming harmful pathogens.
- **Cross-Contamination Awareness**: The Bible's emphasis on separating clean and unclean animals can be seen as an early form of understanding cross-contamination. Modern food safety practices stress the importance of preventing cross-contamination to avoid spreading pathogens from raw to cooked foods.

Hygiene:

- **Sanitary Slaughter Practices**: The dietary laws likely promoted more sanitary slaughter and handling practices. For example, animals that chew the cud are less likely to consume waste or carrion, reducing the risk of contaminating meat with harmful bacteria.

- **Avoidance of Scavengers**: Many of the unclean birds and animals are scavengers, consuming dead animals and waste, which increases their likelihood of carrying diseases. By avoiding these creatures, the Israelites minimized their exposure to potential health hazards.

Modern Dietary Practices:

- **Healthy Eating Patterns**: Emphasizing clean animals and avoiding unclean ones can guide modern dietary choices toward healthier eating patterns. For example, choosing lean meats, fish with fins and scales, and poultry aligns with contemporary recommendations for a balanced diet.

- **Environmental Considerations**: The principles in Leviticus 11 can also inform environmentally sustainable eating practices. Consuming plant-based foods and clean animals raised in humane and sustainable ways can reduce the environmental impact of our diets.

Scientific Validation:

- **Supporting Research**: Modern research supports many of the health benefits associated with the clean foods described in Leviticus 11. Studies have shown that diets rich in fish, lean meats, and plant-based foods are associated with lower risks of chronic diseases such as heart disease, diabetes, and cancer.

- **Understanding Allergens and Toxins**: Shellfish and certain fish are common allergens and can accumulate toxins like mercury, which pose significant health risks. The biblical prohibition of these foods aligns with modern understanding of food allergens and toxins.

Integrating Biblical Principles with Modern Nutrition

Integrating the principles of clean and unclean foods from Leviticus 11 with modern nutrition involves understanding the wisdom behind these ancient guidelines and applying them in ways that enhance contemporary health practices.

Balanced Diet:

- **Whole Foods Emphasis**: Embrace a diet rich in whole, unprocessed foods, including fruits, vegetables, whole grains, and lean proteins. This approach mirrors the biblical emphasis on consuming foods that are pure and natural.

- **Moderation and Variety**: Practice moderation and include a variety of foods in your diet to ensure a wide range of nutrients. This aligns with the biblical principle of balance and avoiding excess.

Mindful Eating:

- **Gratitude and Mindfulness**: Approach eating with gratitude and mindfulness, recognizing food as a gift from God. This perspective encourages a healthier relationship with food and promotes mindful eating practices.

- **Fasting and Spiritual Health**: Incorporate fasting into your routine as a way to enhance spiritual health and promote physical well-being. Fasting has been shown to have numerous health benefits, including improved metabolism and mental clarity.

Sustainable and Ethical Choices:

- **Environmental Stewardship**: Make dietary choices that reflect a commitment to environmental stewardship. Opt for sustainably sourced fish, organic produce, and humanely raised meats. This practice aligns with the biblical call to care for God's creation.

- **Ethical Considerations**: Consider the ethical implications of your food choices, including the treatment of animals and the impact on local communities. Choose foods that promote justice and compassion, reflecting biblical values.

The dietary laws outlined in Leviticus 11 offer timeless wisdom that continues to resonate in the modern world. By understanding the principles of clean and unclean foods, we can make informed dietary choices that promote health, safety, and spiritual well-being. Integrating these biblical guidelines with contemporary nutritional science enhances our ability to live healthy, balanced lives that honor God and His creation.

As we navigate the complexities of modern diets and food systems, let us remember the wisdom of the Scriptures and strive to make choices that reflect both our faith and our commitment to health. By embracing the principles of clean and unclean foods, we can experience the holistic benefits of a diet that is both nourishing and spiritually enriching.

Chapter 3: Feasting and Fasting in the Bible

Matthew 4:2 – "And when he had fasted forty days and forty nights, he was afterward an hungred."

Fasting is a practice deeply rooted in biblical tradition, serving both physical and spiritual purposes. Matthew 4:2 recounts Jesus' 40-day fast in the wilderness, a period of intense spiritual preparation and physical challenge. This act of fasting is emblematic of the dual nature of fasting: it serves as a profound spiritual discipline and offers significant physical benefits.

Importance of Fasting for Physical and Spiritual Health

Spiritual Significance of Fasting

Fasting, in the biblical context, is more than abstaining from food; it is a powerful spiritual discipline that draws believers closer to God. The Bible is replete with examples of fasting as a means of seeking divine guidance, repentance, and spiritual strength.

1. **Seeking God's Guidance**:

- In Acts 13:2-3, we see the early church fasting and praying before making significant decisions. "While they were worshiping the Lord and fasting, the Holy Spirit said, 'Set apart for me Barnabas and Saul for the work to which I have called them.' So after they had fasted and prayed, they placed their hands on them and sent them off."
- Fasting helps believers to focus on spiritual matters, creating an environment conducive to hearing God's voice more clearly.

1. **Repentance and Humility**:

- Fasting is often associated with repentance and seeking God's mercy. In the book of Jonah, the people of Nineveh proclaimed a fast and put on sackcloth as a sign of their repentance (Jonah 3:5).
- It serves as a physical manifestation of inner humility and contrition, aligning the body with the heart's intent to seek forgiveness and renewal.

1. **Spiritual Warfare and Strength**:

- Jesus' 40-day fast in the wilderness (Matthew 4:1-11) was a period of spiritual preparation before beginning His public ministry. This fast was marked by intense spiritual warfare, as Jesus resisted Satan's temptations through the power of the Spirit and the Word.
- Fasting strengthens the believer's resolve and dependence on God, equipping them for spiritual battles and ministry.

Physical Health Benefits of Fasting

While fasting is primarily a spiritual discipline, it also offers numerous physical health benefits that are increasingly recognized by modern science. These benefits include improved metabolic health, enhanced brain function, and increased longevity.

1. **Improved Metabolic Health**:

- Fasting helps to regulate blood sugar levels, improve insulin sensitivity, and reduce the risk of type 2 diabetes. A study published in the journal Cell Metabolism found that intermittent fasting can lead to significant improvements in metabolic health markers.
- By giving the digestive system regular breaks, fasting allows the body to reset and repair, promoting better overall metabolic function.

1. **Enhanced Brain Function**:

- Fasting has been shown to stimulate the production of brain-derived neurotrophic factor (BDNF), a protein that supports neuron growth and cognitive function. According to research published in the Journal of Neuroscience, increased BDNF levels can enhance memory and learning.
- Additionally, fasting may reduce inflammation and oxidative stress in the brain, protecting against neurodegenerative diseases like Alzheimer's and Parkinson's.

1. **Increased Longevity**:

- Studies on various organisms, from yeast to mammals, have demonstrated that caloric restriction and fasting can extend lifespan. Research published in Nature Communications suggests that intermittent fasting can promote cellular repair processes and reduce markers of aging.

- Fasting triggers autophagy, a cellular cleaning process that removes damaged cells and regenerates new ones, contributing to longevity and overall health.

Modern Relevance: Intermittent Fasting and Its Health Benefits

Intermittent fasting (IF) is a modern approach to fasting that mirrors many biblical principles and has gained popularity for its health benefits. IF involves cycling between periods of eating and fasting, with various methods such as the 16/8 (fasting for 16 hours and eating within an 8-hour window) or the 5:2 (eating normally for five days and reducing calorie intake for two non-consecutive days).

Scientific Support for Intermittent Fasting

1. **Weight Management**:

- IF is effective for weight loss and weight management. By restricting the eating window, IF naturally reduces calorie intake without the need for strict dieting. A review in the Annual Review of Nutrition found that IF can lead to significant reductions in body weight and fat mass.
- The body's metabolism adjusts to fasting periods by using stored fat for energy, promoting fat loss while preserving lean muscle mass.

1. **Cardiovascular Health**:

- IF can improve cardiovascular health by reducing blood pressure, cholesterol levels, and inflammatory markers. A study in the British Journal of Nutrition reported that IF participants showed improved lipid profiles and lower blood pressure.

- Fasting periods allow the cardiovascular system to rest and repair, reducing the risk of heart disease and stroke.

1. **Mental Clarity and Emotional Well-being**:

- Many individuals report increased mental clarity and improved mood during fasting periods. IF can stabilize blood sugar levels, preventing the energy crashes that often lead to irritability and poor concentration.
- The practice of fasting, with its discipline and routine, can also provide a sense of accomplishment and emotional stability, contributing to better mental health.

Integrating Biblical Fasting with Intermittent Fasting

Combining the spiritual discipline of biblical fasting with the health benefits of intermittent fasting offers a holistic approach to well-being. Here are some practical ways to integrate these practices into daily life:

1. **Start with Prayer and Intention**:

- Begin your fast with prayer, seeking God's guidance and dedicating your fasting period to a specific spiritual purpose. Whether it's seeking clarity, interceding for others, or deepening your relationship with God, set a clear intention for your fast.

1. **Choose a Fasting Method**:

- Select an intermittent fasting method that suits your lifestyle. The 16/8 method is a popular choice for beginners, as it allows for a manageable fasting period while providing ample time for nourishment.

- Align your fasting schedule with your spiritual practices. For example, you might choose to fast from dinner to lunch the next day, using the morning hours for prayer and meditation.

1. **Stay Hydrated and Nourished**:

- During fasting periods, stay hydrated with water, herbal teas, and broths. Proper hydration supports your body's detoxification processes and maintains energy levels.
- When breaking your fast, choose nutrient-dense foods that nourish your body and support your spiritual goals. Focus on whole, unprocessed foods rich in vitamins, minerals, and antioxidants.

1. **Embrace the Spiritual Journey**:

- Use fasting as an opportunity to disconnect from distractions and focus on your spiritual growth. Spend time in prayer, reading Scripture, and reflecting on your faith journey.
- Fasting can reveal areas of your life that need transformation, allowing the Holy Spirit to work in and through you. Embrace this process with an open heart and mind.

1. **Reflect and Record Your Experience**:

- Keep a journal to document your fasting experience, noting any physical, emotional, and spiritual insights. Reflecting on your journey can provide valuable insights and encourage continued growth.
- Share your experiences with a trusted community or spiritual mentor. Accountability and support can enhance your fasting practice and deepen your spiritual connections.

The practice of fasting, as demonstrated in the Bible and supported by modern science, offers a profound means of enhancing both physical health and spiritual well-being. By understanding the importance of fasting for physical and spiritual health, we can embrace this discipline with renewed purpose and intentionality.

Intermittent fasting provides a practical framework for integrating fasting into our modern lives, offering numerous health benefits while aligning with biblical principles. Whether seeking God's guidance, repenting, or preparing for spiritual warfare, fasting serves as a powerful tool for drawing closer to God and enhancing our overall well-being.

As we embark on the journey of fasting, let us do so with a heart of humility, gratitude, and faith. May our fasting periods be times of deep spiritual renewal and physical rejuvenation, reflecting the holistic nature of our Creator's design for health and wholeness.

Part 2: Biblical Diet for Diabetes

Chapter 4. Diabetes in Biblical Context

Diabetes, a chronic condition characterized by elevated blood sugar levels, is one of the most prevalent and serious health issues facing the modern world. Understanding diabetes from a biblical context involves exploring how ancient wisdom aligns with contemporary scientific understanding and how biblical principles can inform modern dietary practices to manage and prevent this condition.

Diabetes occurs when the body either does not produce enough insulin or cannot effectively use the insulin it produces. This leads to elevated levels of glucose in the blood, which can cause a range of health problems, including heart disease, nerve damage, kidney failure, and vision loss. The two main types of diabetes are Type 1, which is often diagnosed in childhood and involves the immune system attacking insulin-producing cells in the pancreas, and Type 2, which is more common and typically develops in adults as a result of insulin resistance.

The prevalence of diabetes has skyrocketed in recent decades, with the World Health Organization (WHO) reporting that the number of people with diabetes has nearly quadrupled since 1980. This increase is largely driven by lifestyle factors such as poor diet, physical inactivity, and obesity. However, the wisdom found in biblical teachings offers timeless guidance that can help mitigate these risk factors and manage diabetes effectively.

Proverbs 25:16 – "Have you found honey? Eat only as much as you need, Lest you be filled with it and vomit."

This proverb, while seemingly simple, encapsulates a profound principle of moderation that is crucial for managing diabetes. Honey, a natural source of sugar, is used metaphorically here to represent all forms of sweetness and pleasure. The admonition to eat only as much as needed speaks directly to the dangers of overconsumption, particularly of sugary foods and beverages, which are major contributors to the development and exacerbation of diabetes.

Moderation in Sugar Intake

Moderation is a key biblical principle that is highly relevant in the context of diabetes management. The excessive consumption of sugar and refined carbohydrates is a major risk factor for developing Type 2 diabetes. This is because these foods cause rapid spikes in blood sugar levels, leading to insulin resistance over time.

The modern diet is replete with hidden sugars and refined carbohydrates found in processed foods, sugary drinks, and snacks. These foods not only contribute to weight gain and obesity, which are major risk factors for diabetes, but also lead to metabolic dysfunctions that impair the body's ability to regulate blood sugar.

Biblical Principles for Modern Dietary Practices

1. **Natural, Whole Foods**:

    o   The Bible emphasizes the consumption of natural, whole foods, which are inherently nutrient-dense and free from the harmful additives found in processed foods. Genesis 1:29 highlights God's provision of plants and fruits for food, underscoring the health benefits of a diet rich in vegetables, fruits, nuts, seeds, and whole grains.

    o   Modern science supports this, showing that diets high in whole foods help maintain stable blood sugar levels, reduce inflammation, and improve overall metabolic health. Foods high in fiber, such as vegetables and whole grains, slow the absorption of sugar into the bloodstream, preventing spikes in blood glucose levels.

1. **Balanced Diet**:

    o   A balanced diet that includes a variety of nutrients is essential for managing diabetes. The Mediterranean diet, which closely resembles biblical dietary patterns, is rich in fruits, vegetables, whole grains, fish, and olive oil. This diet has been shown to improve blood sugar control and reduce the risk of diabetes-related complications.

    o   Proverbs 15:17 states, "Better is a dinner of herbs where love is, than a fattened ox and hatred with it." This emphasizes the value of simple, wholesome meals over rich, indulgent foods, aligning with modern recommendations to prioritize plant-based foods and lean proteins over high-fat, high-sugar options.

1. **Portion Control**:

- Proverbs 25:16's emphasis on moderation is a call to be mindful of portion sizes. Overeating, even of healthy foods, can lead to weight gain and metabolic imbalances. Practicing portion control helps maintain a healthy weight and prevents overloading the body with excess calories and sugars.
- The concept of mindful eating, which involves paying full attention to the experience of eating and drinking, is rooted in biblical principles of gratitude and awareness. By being mindful of what and how much we eat, we can make healthier choices that support diabetes management.

1. **Regular Fasting**:

- Fasting is a common biblical practice that has significant health benefits, including improved insulin sensitivity and weight loss. Intermittent fasting, which involves cycling between periods of eating and fasting, can help regulate blood sugar levels and reduce the risk of diabetes.
- Jesus' 40-day fast in the wilderness (Matthew 4:2) exemplifies the spiritual and physical benefits of fasting. Modern research supports intermittent fasting as a beneficial practice for metabolic health, showing that it can lower blood sugar levels, reduce insulin resistance, and promote weight loss.

1. **Healthy Fats and Proteins**:

- The Bible includes references to consuming healthy fats and proteins, such as olive oil and fish. These foods are essential for maintaining stable blood sugar levels and providing sustained energy. Omega-3 fatty acids, found in fish like salmon and mackerel, are particularly beneficial for reducing inflammation and improving insulin sensitivity.

- In contrast, the Bible warns against excessive consumption of rich, fatty foods. For example, Proverbs 23:20-21 advises, "Do not join those who drink too much wine or gorge themselves on meat, for drunkards and gluttons become poor, and drowsiness clothes them in rags." This aligns with modern advice to limit saturated fats and trans fats, which can contribute to insulin resistance and cardiovascular disease.

1. **Hydration and Avoiding Sugary Drinks**:

- Proper hydration is emphasized in the Bible and is crucial for managing diabetes. Drinking water instead of sugary beverages helps maintain healthy blood sugar levels. Proverbs 25:25 says, "Like cold water to a weary soul is good news from a distant land," highlighting the refreshing and life-sustaining quality of water.
- Sugary drinks, including sodas and fruit juices, are major contributors to excess sugar intake and should be avoided. These beverages cause rapid spikes in blood sugar levels and provide little to no nutritional value. Instead, drinking water, herbal teas, and other non-sugary beverages supports overall health and hydration.

Practical Steps to Implement a Biblical Diet for Diabetes

1. **Increase Fiber Intake**:

- Incorporate more high-fiber foods into your diet, such as vegetables, fruits, legumes, and whole grains. Fiber slows the absorption of sugar into the bloodstream, helping to maintain stable blood sugar levels.
- Example: Start your day with a bowl of oatmeal topped with fresh berries and a sprinkle of flaxseeds. Include a side salad with a variety of colorful vegetables with your lunch and dinner.

1. **Choose Whole Grains**:

    ◦ Replace refined grains with whole grains like brown rice, quinoa, barley, and whole-wheat products. Whole grains have a lower glycemic index, meaning they have a slower, more gradual effect on blood sugar levels.

    ◦ Example: Substitute white rice with brown rice or quinoa in your meals. Choose whole-grain bread and pasta over their refined counterparts.

2. **Incorporate Healthy Proteins and Fats**:

    ◦ Include lean proteins and healthy fats in your meals to promote satiety and stabilize blood sugar levels. Examples include fish, poultry, nuts, seeds, and olive oil.

    ◦ Example: Enjoy a grilled salmon fillet with a side of steamed vegetables and a drizzle of olive oil. Snack on a handful of almonds or a small serving of Greek yogurt with chia seeds.

3. **Practice Portion Control**:

    ◦ Be mindful of portion sizes to avoid overeating. Use smaller plates and bowls to help control portions and avoid second helpings.

    ◦ Example: Serve meals on smaller plates and take the time to savor each bite. Pay attention to hunger and fullness cues to avoid eating out of habit or boredom.

4. **Stay Hydrated**:

    ◦ Drink plenty of water throughout the day to stay hydrated and support overall health. Avoid sugary drinks and opt for water, herbal teas, or infused water with slices of citrus or cucumber.

    ◦ Example: Carry a reusable water bottle with you and aim to drink at least eight 8-ounce glasses of water each day. Replace sugary drinks with sparkling water flavored with a splash of lemon or lime juice.

1. **Plan and Prepare Meals**:

- Plan your meals and snacks ahead of time to ensure you have healthy options readily available. Meal prepping can help you stay on track with your dietary goals and avoid the temptation of unhealthy foods.
- Example: Dedicate one day each week to meal planning and preparation. Cook and portion out meals in advance, so you have nutritious options ready to go during busy days.

1. **Regular Physical Activity**:

- Incorporate regular physical activity into your routine to help manage blood sugar levels and improve overall health. Exercise enhances insulin sensitivity and aids in weight management.
- Example: Aim for at least 150 minutes of moderate-intensity aerobic activity each week, such as brisk walking, cycling, or swimming. Include strength training exercises at least two days a week.

The biblical principles of moderation, natural whole foods, balanced diet, portion control, regular fasting, healthy fats and proteins, and hydration offer a comprehensive framework for managing and preventing diabetes. By integrating these timeless principles with modern scientific understanding, we can develop effective dietary strategies that promote health and well-being.

Proverbs 25:16's call for moderation in sugar intake is particularly relevant in today's world, where overconsumption of sugary foods and beverages is rampant. By embracing a biblical diet, individuals can achieve better blood sugar control, reduce the risk of diabetes-related complications, and improve overall health.

As a Christian preacher and seasoned nutritionist, I encourage you to reflect on the wisdom found in Scripture and apply these principles to your daily life. By making mindful, informed dietary choices, we honor our bodies as temples of the Holy Spirit and promote physical, spiritual, and emotional well-being. Let us seek God's guidance in our dietary practices and trust in His provision for our health and vitality.

Chapter 5: Foods to Include

Whole Grains, Legumes, Nuts, and Seeds

The Bible, in its timeless wisdom, emphasizes the importance of wholesome, natural foods. Whole grains, legumes, nuts, and seeds are not only biblically endorsed but also scientifically proven to be beneficial for health, particularly in managing blood sugar levels. This chapter explores the biblical basis for these foods, their health benefits, and their modern relevance, particularly focusing on their low glycemic index (GI) and impact on blood sugar levels.

Biblical Basis for Whole Grains, Legumes, Nuts, and Seeds

The consumption of whole grains, legumes, nuts, and seeds is deeply rooted in biblical teachings. These foods were staples in the diet of ancient Israel and are frequently mentioned throughout the Scriptures.

1. **Whole Grains**:

- **Genesis 1:29**: "And God said, Behold, I have given you every herb bearing seed, which is upon the face of all the earth, and every tree, in the which is the fruit of a tree yielding seed; to you it shall be for meat."
- **Ezekiel 4:9**: "Take also unto thee wheat, and barley, and beans, and lentils, and millet, and spelt, and put them in one vessel, and make thee bread thereof."
- Whole grains such as wheat, barley, and millet were central to the diet of the Israelites. Ezekiel's bread, made from a variety of grains and legumes, highlights the nutritional diversity and balance inherent in their diet.

1. **Legumes**:

- **2 Samuel 17:28-29**: "Brought beds, and basins, and earthen vessels, and wheat, and barley, and flour, and parched corn, and beans, and lentils, and parched pulse, And honey, and butter, and sheep, and cheese of kine, for David, and for the people that were with him, to eat."
- Legumes like beans and lentils were valuable sources of protein and nutrients, often included in meals for their sustenance and health benefits.

1. **Nuts and Seeds**:

- **Genesis 43:11**: "Then their father Israel said to them, 'If it must be so, then do this: take some of the choice fruits of the land in your bags, and carry down a present to the man, a little balm and a little honey, gum, myrrh, pistachio nuts, and almonds.'"

o   Nuts and seeds, such as pistachios and almonds, were considered delicacies and important food sources, providing essential fats, protein, and vitamins.

Modern Relevance: Low Glycemic Index Foods and Their Impact on Blood Sugar Levels

The concept of the glycemic index (GI) is crucial in understanding how foods impact blood sugar levels. The GI measures how quickly carbohydrates in food are converted into glucose in the bloodstream. Foods with a low GI release glucose more slowly and steadily, which helps maintain stable blood sugar levels and reduces the risk of insulin spikes.

Whole Grains

Health Benefits:

- **Nutrient-Rich**: Whole grains retain all parts of the grain kernel – the bran, germ, and endosperm. This means they are rich in fiber, vitamins (such as B vitamins), minerals (such as iron, magnesium, and selenium), and antioxidants.
- **Heart Health**: Consumption of whole grains is linked to a lower risk of heart disease. The fiber in whole grains helps reduce cholesterol levels, while antioxidants protect against heart disease.
- **Digestive Health**: The high fiber content in whole grains promotes healthy digestion, prevents constipation, and supports a healthy gut microbiome.

Low GI and Blood Sugar Control:

- Whole grains like barley, oats, quinoa, and brown rice have a low to moderate GI, meaning they cause a slower, more gradual rise in blood sugar levels. This is beneficial for managing diabetes and preventing blood sugar spikes.
- For example, barley has a GI of 28, while quinoa's GI ranges from 53 to 57. These grains provide sustained energy and help maintain satiety, reducing the likelihood of overeating.

Practical Tips:

- **Incorporate into Meals**: Start your day with a bowl of oatmeal topped with nuts and seeds. Use quinoa or brown rice as a base for salads and main dishes. Swap refined grains for whole grain alternatives in recipes.
- **Cooking Methods**: Soak grains overnight to reduce cooking time and improve digestibility. Experiment with different grains to add variety and nutritional diversity to your diet.

Legumes

Health Benefits:

- **High in Protein and Fiber**: Legumes are excellent sources of plant-based protein and dietary fiber, which help regulate digestion and support muscle health.
- **Rich in Vitamins and Minerals**: They provide essential nutrients such as folate, iron, magnesium, and potassium, which are important for overall health.
- **Low in Fat**: Legumes are naturally low in fat and contain no cholesterol, making them heart-healthy choices.

Low GI and Blood Sugar Control:

- Legumes have a low GI, making them ideal for managing blood sugar levels. For example, lentils have a GI of around 32, while chickpeas have a GI of 28.
- The high fiber and protein content in legumes slows the digestion process and the absorption of glucose, leading to a more stable blood sugar response.

Practical Tips:
- **Versatile Use**: Add beans and lentils to soups, stews, and salads. Use them as a base for vegetarian burgers and spreads.
- **Preparation**: Soak dried beans overnight to reduce cooking time and improve digestibility. Rinse canned beans thoroughly to remove excess sodium.

Nuts and Seeds

Health Benefits:
- **Rich in Healthy Fats**: Nuts and seeds are high in monounsaturated and polyunsaturated fats, which are beneficial for heart health.
- **High in Protein and Fiber**: They provide a good amount of protein and fiber, promoting satiety and supporting muscle health.
- **Packed with Micronutrients**: Nuts and seeds are rich in vitamins and minerals such as vitamin E, magnesium, zinc, and selenium, which are essential for various bodily functions.

Low GI and Blood Sugar Control:
- Nuts and seeds have a minimal impact on blood sugar levels due to their low carbohydrate content and high fat and fiber content. This makes them excellent choices for managing diabetes and preventing blood sugar spikes.
- For example, almonds have a GI of 0, meaning they do not cause a significant rise in blood sugar levels.

Practical Tips:

- **Incorporate into Meals and Snacks**: Add a handful of nuts to your breakfast cereal or yogurt. Use nut butters as spreads or in smoothies. Sprinkle seeds over salads, soups, and baked goods.
- **Portion Control**: While nuts and seeds are nutritious, they are also calorie-dense. Be mindful of portion sizes to avoid excessive calorie intake.

Integrating Whole Grains, Legumes, Nuts, and Seeds into a Balanced Diet

1. **Meal Planning**:

    - Plan your meals to include a variety of whole grains, legumes, nuts, and seeds. This ensures a balanced intake of essential nutrients and keeps your diet interesting.
    - Example: A day's meal plan might include oatmeal with nuts and seeds for breakfast, a quinoa salad with chickpeas and vegetables for lunch, and a lentil stew with brown rice for dinner.

1. **Healthy Snacking**:

    - Keep nuts and seeds on hand for quick and healthy snacks. Pair them with fresh fruit or yogurt for a balanced snack that provides protein, healthy fats, and fiber.
    - Example: Snack on a small handful of almonds and an apple in the afternoon to keep your energy levels stable.

1. **Experiment with Recipes**:

    - Try new recipes that feature whole grains, legumes, nuts, and seeds. Explore different cuisines that traditionally use these foods, such as Mediterranean, Middle Eastern, and Indian dishes.

- Example: Make a batch of homemade hummus using chickpeas, tahini (sesame seed paste), lemon juice, and garlic. Enjoy it with whole grain pita bread or vegetable sticks.

1. **Mindful Eating**:

- Practice mindful eating by paying attention to your hunger and fullness cues. Enjoy the textures, flavors, and aromas of whole grains, legumes, nuts, and seeds.
- Example: Take the time to savor a bowl of quinoa salad, noticing the crunch of the vegetables and the nutty flavor of the quinoa.

1. **Combining Foods for Synergy**:

- Combine whole grains, legumes, nuts, and seeds in meals to maximize nutritional benefits and enhance flavor. The combination of protein, fiber, and healthy fats helps maintain stable blood sugar levels and promotes satiety.
- Example: Create a power bowl with a base of brown rice, topped with black beans, avocado slices, and a sprinkle of pumpkin seeds. Drizzle with olive oil and a squeeze of lime for added flavor and nutrition.

The inclusion of whole grains, legumes, nuts, and seeds in the diet aligns with both biblical wisdom and modern scientific understanding. These foods are nutrient-dense, support stable blood sugar levels, and provide a range of health benefits that are crucial for managing diabetes and promoting overall well-being.

By integrating these foods into your diet, you can create balanced, satisfying meals that nourish your body and support your health. Embracing the principles of moderation, variety, and mindful eating, as taught in the Bible, helps you maintain a healthy relationship with food and honors the divine wisdom of caring for your body.

As a Christian preacher and seasoned nutritionist, I encourage you to reflect on the timeless teachings of Scripture and apply them to your dietary choices. By doing so, you can achieve better health, prevent and manage diabetes, and enjoy the abundant life that God intends for you. Let us give thanks for the bounty of nutritious foods provided by our Creator and commit to making choices that honor both our bodies and our faith.

Chapter 6: Foods to Avoid

Excessive Sugars and Refined Carbohydrates

The Bible provides timeless wisdom regarding the consumption of foods and the importance of moderation. In modern times, understanding and applying these biblical principles can guide us in making healthier dietary choices. This chapter explores the biblical perspective on excessive sugars and refined carbohydrates, their impact on health, and the modern relevance of avoiding processed foods and sugary drinks.

Biblical Perspective on Excessive Sugars and Refined Carbohydrates

1. **Moderation and Self-Control**:

    o **Proverbs 25:16**: "Have you found honey? Eat only as much as you need, Lest you be filled with it and vomit."

- This proverb teaches the principle of moderation, emphasizing the need to avoid overconsumption, even of good things like honey, which represents natural sugars. The wisdom here is clear: consuming excessive amounts of sugar can lead to negative consequences.

1. **Guarding Against Gluttony**:

   - **Philippians 3:19**: "Their end is destruction, their god is their belly, and they glory in their shame, with minds set on earthly things."
   - The Bible warns against gluttony, which can be interpreted as overindulgence in any food, including sugars and refined carbohydrates. The spiritual discipline of self-control is essential for maintaining both physical and spiritual health.

1. **The Body as a Temple**:

   - **1 Corinthians 6:19-20**: "Do you not know that your bodies are temples of the Holy Spirit, who is in you, whom you have received from God? You are not your own; you were bought at a price. Therefore honor God with your bodies."
   - This passage highlights the importance of taking care of our bodies as temples of the Holy Spirit. Consuming excessive sugars and refined carbohydrates can harm our health, thus dishonoring the temple that God has entrusted to us.

The Impact of Excessive Sugars and Refined Carbohydrates on Health

Excessive consumption of sugars and refined carbohydrates is linked to a multitude of health issues. These include obesity, type 2 diabetes, heart disease, and metabolic syndrome. Understanding the science behind these impacts can help us appreciate the wisdom of biblical dietary principles.

1. **Obesity and Weight Gain:**

    o   Sugars and refined carbohydrates are calorie-dense but nutrient-poor. They contribute to excessive calorie intake without providing the essential nutrients needed for health. This can lead to weight gain and obesity, which are significant risk factors for many chronic diseases.

    o   **Scientific Evidence**: A study published in the American Journal of Clinical Nutrition found that diets high in sugar-sweetened beverages were associated with increased body weight and obesity.

1. **Type 2 Diabetes:**

    o   High intake of sugars and refined carbohydrates causes rapid spikes in blood sugar levels, leading to insulin resistance over time. This is a primary factor in the development of type 2 diabetes.

    o   **Scientific Evidence**: Research in the journal Diabetes Care highlights that excessive consumption of sugar-sweetened beverages increases the risk of developing type 2 diabetes by contributing to insulin resistance and beta-cell dysfunction.

1. **Heart Disease:**

    o   Diets high in sugars and refined carbohydrates can lead to increased levels of triglycerides, LDL (bad) cholesterol, and inflammation, all of which are risk factors for heart disease.

    o   **Scientific Evidence**: A study in the Journal of the American Heart Association found that high sugar intake is associated with an increased risk of cardiovascular disease mortality.

1. **Metabolic Syndrome:**

    o   Metabolic syndrome is a cluster of conditions, including increased blood pressure, high blood sugar, excess body fat around the waist, and abnormal cholesterol levels. High intake of refined carbohydrates and sugars is a significant contributing factor.

- **Scientific Evidence**: Research in the journal Circulation has shown that diets high in refined carbohydrates and sugars increase the risk of developing metabolic syndrome.

Modern Relevance: The Dangers of Processed Foods and Sugary Drinks

In today's world, processed foods and sugary drinks are ubiquitous. Understanding their dangers and learning to avoid them is crucial for maintaining good health.

1. **Processed Foods**:

- Processed foods are often high in added sugars, unhealthy fats, and sodium. They are also typically low in essential nutrients such as fiber, vitamins, and minerals. Consuming these foods regularly can lead to various health issues.
- **Examples**: Examples of processed foods include snack cakes, cookies, breakfast cereals, and fast food items. These foods often contain high-fructose corn syrup, trans fats, and artificial additives.

1. **Sugary Drinks**:

- Sugary drinks, including sodas, fruit juices, and energy drinks, are significant sources of added sugars in the diet. They provide empty calories without any nutritional benefits and contribute to the risk of obesity, diabetes, and other chronic diseases.
- **Examples**: Regular soda, sweetened iced tea, lemonade, and many commercially available fruit juices and sports drinks are loaded with sugars.

Health Impacts:

- **Weight Gain and Obesity**: Sugary drinks contribute significantly to weight gain due to their high sugar content and low satiety value. This can lead to an increased risk of obesity-related diseases.
- **Type 2 Diabetes**: The rapid absorption of sugars from sugary drinks causes spikes in blood sugar and insulin levels, increasing the risk of insulin resistance and type 2 diabetes.
- **Dental Problems**: Sugary drinks are a major cause of tooth decay and cavities. The high sugar content provides food for bacteria in the mouth, leading to acid production and tooth enamel erosion.

Practical Steps to Avoid Excessive Sugars and Refined Carbohydrates

1. **Read Food Labels**:

    - **Identify Hidden Sugars**: Many processed foods contain hidden sugars listed under various names, such as high-fructose corn syrup, sucrose, glucose, and maltose. Reading labels carefully helps in identifying and avoiding these hidden sugars.
    - **Choose Whole Foods**: Opt for whole, unprocessed foods whenever possible. Fresh fruits, vegetables, whole grains, and lean proteins should be the foundation of your diet.

1. **Cook at Home**:

    - **Control Ingredients**: Cooking at home allows you to control the ingredients in your meals, reducing the likelihood of consuming added sugars and unhealthy fats.
    - **Healthy Recipes**: Experiment with healthy recipes that use whole grains, legumes, nuts, and seeds. This not only improves nutrition but also enhances the flavor and enjoyment of meals.

1. **Healthy Substitutes**:

- **Natural Sweeteners**: Replace refined sugars with natural sweeteners like honey, maple syrup, or stevia. Use these in moderation to add sweetness without the negative health impacts of refined sugars.
- **Whole Grains**: Substitute refined grains with whole grains such as brown rice, quinoa, barley, and whole-wheat products. These provide more nutrients and fiber, helping to maintain stable blood sugar levels.

1. **Hydrate Wisely**:

- **Water First**: Make water your primary beverage. Add slices of fruit or herbs for flavor if needed. Herbal teas and infused water are also good options.
- **Limit Sugary Drinks**: Avoid sugary drinks and opt for healthier alternatives. If you crave something sweet, try making a smoothie with fresh fruits and a source of protein, such as Greek yogurt or a handful of nuts.

1. **Mindful Eating**:

- **Awareness and Moderation**: Practice mindful eating by being aware of your food choices and the portion sizes you consume. Focus on the quality and nutritional value of the foods you eat.
- **Savor Your Food**: Take the time to savor each bite, enjoying the flavors and textures of whole, natural foods. This practice can reduce the desire for overly sweet or processed foods.

1. **Plan and Prepare**:

- **Meal Prep**: Plan and prepare meals ahead of time to ensure you have healthy options available. This reduces the temptation to choose processed foods or sugary snacks when you are hungry.

- **Balanced Meals**: Ensure each meal includes a balance of macronutrients: proteins, fats, and carbohydrates. This helps maintain energy levels and prevents blood sugar spikes.

The biblical principles of moderation, self-control, and honoring the body as a temple align perfectly with modern scientific understanding of the health impacts of excessive sugars and refined carbohydrates. By avoiding these foods, we can reduce the risk of obesity, type 2 diabetes, heart disease, and other chronic conditions.

The dangers of processed foods and sugary drinks cannot be overstated. These products are major contributors to the current epidemic of chronic diseases. By making informed dietary choices and prioritizing whole, unprocessed foods, we can protect our health and honor God with our bodies.

As a Christian preacher and seasoned nutritionist, I encourage you to reflect on the wisdom found in Scripture and apply these principles to your dietary choices. By doing so, you can achieve better health, prevent disease, and enjoy the abundant life that God intends for you. Let us seek God's guidance in our dietary practices and trust in His provision for our health and vitality.

Part 3: Biblical Diet for High Blood Pressure

Chapter 7: High Blood Pressure in Biblical Context

High blood pressure, also known as hypertension, is a prevalent and serious health condition that significantly increases the risk of heart disease, stroke, and kidney disease. It is often referred to as a "silent killer" because it typically has no symptoms until significant damage has occurred. Understanding the biblical context of dietary practices can offer valuable insights into managing and preventing high blood pressure through natural means, particularly emphasizing a plant-based diet.

Explanation of Hypertension

Hypertension is a condition in which the force of the blood against the artery walls is consistently too high. Blood pressure is measured in millimeters of mercury (mm Hg) and is recorded with two numbers: systolic pressure (the top number) measures the pressure in the arteries when the heart beats, and diastolic pressure (the bottom number) measures the pressure in the arteries when the heart is at rest between beats.

Risk Factors for Hypertension:

- **Diet**: High intake of sodium, low intake of potassium, excessive alcohol consumption, and diets high in saturated and trans fats contribute significantly to high blood pressure.
- **Lifestyle**: Lack of physical activity, obesity, smoking, and chronic stress are key risk factors.
- **Genetics**: Family history and age can also play a role in the development of hypertension.

Hypertension is a leading cause of cardiovascular diseases and poses significant health risks, but it can be managed and often prevented through lifestyle changes, particularly diet. The Bible offers timeless wisdom that aligns well with modern nutritional science, providing guidance for a heart-healthy diet.

Daniel 1:12 – "Please test your servants for ten days: Give us nothing but vegetables to eat and water to drink."

The story of Daniel provides a powerful example of the benefits of a plant-based diet. Daniel and his friends, taken captive in Babylon, requested a diet of vegetables and water instead of the king's rich food and wine. After ten days, they appeared healthier and better nourished than those who ate the king's food.

Emphasis on a Plant-Based Diet

Biblical Perspective:

- **Genesis 1:29**: "And God said, Behold, I have given you every herb bearing seed, which is upon the face of all the earth, and every tree, in the which is the fruit of a tree yielding seed; to you it shall be for meat."
  - This verse underscores the original plant-based diet given by God, emphasizing the consumption of fruits, vegetables, seeds, and grains.
- **Proverbs 15:17**: "Better is a dinner of herbs where love is, than a fattened ox and hatred with it."
  - This proverb highlights the value of a simple, plant-based meal over rich, indulgent foods, promoting health and contentment.

Scientific Support for Plant-Based Diets:

1. **Blood Pressure Reduction**:

   - Numerous studies have shown that plant-based diets can significantly reduce blood pressure. Plants are naturally low in sodium and high in potassium, which helps balance blood pressure.
   - **Scientific Evidence**: A study published in the Journal of Hypertension found that individuals who followed a vegetarian diet had significantly lower blood pressure compared to those who consumed meat.

1. **Nutrient-Rich**:

   - Plant-based diets are rich in essential nutrients, including potassium, magnesium, and fiber, all of which play crucial roles in maintaining healthy blood pressure levels.
   - **Potassium**: Helps balance the amount of sodium in cells and is crucial for muscle function, including the heart muscle.
   - **Magnesium**: Involved in over 300 enzymatic reactions in the body, including the regulation of blood pressure.

- **Fiber**: Helps reduce cholesterol levels and improves heart health.

1. **Weight Management**:

- Plant-based diets are typically lower in calories and high in fiber, promoting satiety and helping with weight management, which is crucial for controlling blood pressure.
- **Scientific Evidence**: Research in the American Journal of Clinical Nutrition suggests that plant-based diets are effective for weight loss and maintenance, reducing the risk of hypertension and other cardiovascular diseases.

1. **Anti-Inflammatory Properties**:

- Many plant foods have anti-inflammatory properties that can help reduce inflammation in the blood vessels, improving overall cardiovascular health.
- **Scientific Evidence**: A study in the journal Circulation Research highlights the anti-inflammatory effects of a diet rich in fruits, vegetables, nuts, and seeds.

Practical Application of a Plant-Based Diet for Hypertension

Implementing a plant-based diet can be both simple and rewarding. Here are practical steps and dietary strategies to help manage and prevent high blood pressure.

1. **Incorporate a Variety of Vegetables**:

- Aim to fill half your plate with vegetables at each meal. Include a wide range of colors and types to ensure a diverse intake of nutrients.

- **Examples**: Leafy greens (spinach, kale), cruciferous vegetables (broccoli, cauliflower), root vegetables (carrots, sweet potatoes), and legumes (beans, lentils).

1. **Focus on Fruits**:

- Fruits are rich in potassium, fiber, and antioxidants. Include a variety of fruits in your diet, focusing on whole fruits rather than fruit juices to maximize fiber intake and avoid added sugars.
- **Examples**: Berries, apples, oranges, bananas, and melons.

1. **Choose Whole Grains**:

- Whole grains are an excellent source of fiber, which helps manage blood pressure and improve heart health. Replace refined grains with whole grain alternatives.
- **Examples**: Brown rice, quinoa, barley, oats, whole wheat, and farro.

1. **Include Nuts and Seeds**:

- Nuts and seeds provide healthy fats, protein, and essential nutrients. They can be a great addition to meals or snacks.
- **Examples**: Almonds, walnuts, chia seeds, flaxseeds, and pumpkin seeds.

1. **Limit Sodium Intake**:

- High sodium intake is a major contributor to high blood pressure. Reducing sodium intake can help manage blood pressure effectively.
- **Strategies**: Avoid processed foods, use herbs and spices instead of salt for seasoning, and read food labels to check for sodium content.

1. **Stay Hydrated with Water**:

○ Proper hydration is crucial for maintaining healthy blood pressure levels. Water should be the primary beverage, and sugary drinks should be avoided.

○ **Hydration Tips**: Carry a water bottle, drink a glass of water before meals, and flavor water with slices of citrus or cucumber for variety.

1. **Incorporate Healthy Fats**:

○ Healthy fats from plant sources can help manage blood pressure and improve overall cardiovascular health.

○ **Examples**: Avocados, olive oil, and fatty fish like salmon and mackerel.

Meal Planning and Recipes

Sample Meal Plan:

- **Breakfast**: Oatmeal topped with fresh berries, chia seeds, and a drizzle of almond milk.
- **Lunch**: Quinoa salad with mixed vegetables, chickpeas, and a lemon-tahini dressing.
- **Snack**: A handful of raw almonds and an apple.
- **Dinner**: Stir-fried tofu with broccoli, bell peppers, and brown rice.
- **Dessert**: Fresh fruit salad with a sprinkle of cinnamon.

Recipe: Quinoa Salad with Mixed Vegetables and Chickpeas:

- **Ingredients**:
1. 1 cup quinoa, cooked
2. 1 cup cherry tomatoes, halved
3. 1 cucumber, diced
4. 1 red bell pepper, diced

5. 1 cup chickpeas, drained and rinsed
6. 1/4 cup red onion, finely chopped
7. 2 tbsp fresh parsley, chopped
8. 2 tbsp olive oil
9. Juice of 1 lemon
10. Salt and pepper to taste

- **Instructions**:

1. In a large bowl, combine the cooked quinoa, cherry tomatoes, cucumber, bell pepper, chickpeas, and red onion.
2. In a small bowl, whisk together the olive oil, lemon juice, salt, and pepper.
3. Pour the dressing over the salad and toss to combine.
4. Garnish with fresh parsley and serve.

Recipe: Stir-Fried Tofu with Broccoli and Bell Peppers:

- **Ingredients**:

1. 1 block firm tofu, drained and cubed
2. 1 head of broccoli, cut into florets
3. 1 red bell pepper, sliced
4. 1 yellow bell pepper, sliced
5. 2 cloves garlic, minced
6. 2 tbsp soy sauce (low sodium)
7. 1 tbsp olive oil
8. 1 tsp sesame oil
9. 1 tsp fresh ginger, grated

- **Instructions**:

1. Heat olive oil in a large skillet over medium heat. Add tofu and cook until golden brown on all sides. Remove from skillet and set aside.
2. In the same skillet, add garlic and ginger, and sauté until fragrant.

3. Add broccoli and bell peppers, and cook until tender-crisp.
4. Return tofu to the skillet and add soy sauce and sesame oil. Stir to combine and heat through.
5. Serve over brown rice or quinoa.

The Role of Faith and Community in Health

1. **Spiritual Support**:

   ○ Incorporating faith and prayer into daily life can provide emotional and spiritual support, reducing stress, which is a risk factor for hypertension. Regular prayer and meditation can help cultivate a sense of peace and well-being.

1. **Community and Accountability**:

   ○ Engaging with a faith community can offer encouragement and accountability in making healthy lifestyle choices. Group activities such as communal meals, cooking classes, and walking clubs can promote a plant-based diet and physical activity.

1. **Education and Advocacy**:

   ○ Churches and faith-based organizations can play a crucial role in educating members about the importance of a plant-based diet for managing high blood pressure. Hosting workshops, seminars, and health fairs can disseminate valuable information and resources.

The biblical story of Daniel and his choice of a plant-based diet provides a powerful example of how dietary choices can lead to better health. Emphasizing a plant-based diet is not only biblically sound but also supported by modern scientific research as an effective way to manage and prevent high blood pressure.

By incorporating a variety of vegetables, fruits, whole grains, nuts, and seeds into our diets, and by practicing moderation and mindful eating, we can significantly reduce the risk of hypertension and improve overall health. Additionally, engaging with faith and community support can enhance our commitment to making healthy choices and maintaining a heart-healthy lifestyle.

As a Christian preacher and seasoned nutritionist, I encourage you to embrace the biblical principles of a plant-based diet and apply them to your daily life. By doing so, you can honor your body as a temple of the Holy Spirit, achieve better health, and enjoy the abundant life that God intends for you. Let us seek God's guidance in our dietary practices and trust in His provision for our health and vitality.

CHAPTER 8: FOODS TO INCLUDE

Leafy Greens, Beets, Bananas, and Seeds

The Bible provides timeless principles for maintaining health and well-being, emphasizing the importance of natural, whole foods. Leafy greens, beets, bananas, and seeds are not only biblically endorsed but also scientifically proven to offer significant health benefits, particularly in managing blood pressure. This chapter explores the biblical basis for these foods, their health benefits, and their modern relevance, focusing on their role as potassium-rich foods in blood pressure management.

Biblical Basis for Leafy Greens, Beets, Bananas, and Seeds

The consumption of natural, nutrient-dense foods is deeply rooted in biblical teachings. The Bible frequently references plant-based foods, highlighting their importance for sustenance and health.

1. **Leafy Greens**:

- **Genesis 1:29**: "And God said, Behold, I have given you every herb bearing seed, which is upon the face of all the earth, and every tree, in the which is the fruit of a tree yielding seed; to you it shall be for meat."
- This verse underscores the provision of plant foods, including leafy greens, as essential components of the human diet. Leafy greens such as spinach, kale, and collard greens are nutrient-dense and provide a wealth of health benefits.

1. **Beets**:

- While specific references to beets are not found in the Bible, the general principle of consuming vegetables for health is evident. Beets, with their rich nutrient profile and health benefits, align with the biblical emphasis on natural foods.

1. **Bananas**:

- **Deuteronomy 8:8**: "A land of wheat, and barley, and vines, and fig trees, and pomegranates; a land of oil olive, and honey."
- Although bananas are not specifically mentioned, the inclusion of fruits in the diet is highlighted. Bananas, like figs and pomegranates, are nutritious fruits that contribute to overall health.

1. **Seeds**:

- **Genesis 1:29**: The reference to "every herb bearing seed" includes seeds such as flaxseeds, chia seeds, and pumpkin seeds, which are rich in essential nutrients and beneficial for health.

Health Benefits of Leafy Greens, Beets, Bananas, and Seeds

1. **Leafy Greens**:

    ○   **Nutrient-Dense**: Leafy greens are rich in vitamins A, C, and K, as well as minerals such as iron, calcium, and potassium. They are also high in dietary fiber and antioxidants, which help reduce inflammation and improve overall health.

    ○   **Blood Pressure Management**: Leafy greens are particularly beneficial for managing blood pressure due to their high potassium content. Potassium helps balance sodium levels in the body, reducing the strain on blood vessels and lowering blood pressure.

    ○   **Scientific Evidence**: Research published in the Journal of the American College of Cardiology indicates that increased consumption of leafy greens is associated with a lower risk of cardiovascular diseases, including hypertension.

1. **Beets**:

    ○   **Rich in Nitrates**: Beets are high in dietary nitrates, which the body converts into nitric oxide. Nitric oxide helps relax and dilate blood vessels, improving blood flow and reducing blood pressure.

    ○   **Nutrient Profile**: Beets are also rich in fiber, folate, vitamin C, and potassium, all of which contribute to heart health and blood pressure regulation.

    ○   **Scientific Evidence**: A study in the journal Hypertension found that drinking beet juice significantly lowered blood pressure in hypertensive individuals due to its high nitrate content.

1. **Bananas**:

- **High in Potassium**: Bananas are an excellent source of potassium, which is essential for maintaining proper heart function and regulating blood pressure. One medium-sized banana contains approximately 400-450 mg of potassium.
- **Natural Energy Boost**: Bananas provide a quick source of energy due to their natural sugars and are also high in dietary fiber, which helps regulate blood sugar levels and promotes satiety.
- **Scientific Evidence**: The American Heart Association emphasizes the importance of potassium-rich foods like bananas in managing blood pressure and reducing the risk of stroke.

1. **Seeds**:

- **Nutrient-Rich**: Seeds such as flaxseeds, chia seeds, and pumpkin seeds are rich in omega-3 fatty acids, protein, fiber, and essential minerals like magnesium and potassium. These nutrients support cardiovascular health and help regulate blood pressure.
- **Anti-Inflammatory Properties**: The omega-3 fatty acids in seeds have anti-inflammatory effects that can help reduce blood pressure and improve heart health.
- **Scientific Evidence**: Studies in the journal Nutrition Reviews have shown that the consumption of seeds is associated with improved cardiovascular health and lower blood pressure due to their nutrient density and anti-inflammatory properties.

Modern Relevance: Potassium-Rich Foods and Their Role in Blood Pressure Management

Potassium is a vital mineral that plays a key role in maintaining normal blood pressure. It helps counteract the effects of sodium, relax blood vessel walls, and excrete sodium through urine, thereby reducing blood pressure. Increasing the intake of potassium-rich foods can significantly benefit individuals with hypertension.

Practical Steps to Incorporate Potassium-Rich Foods into the Diet

1. **Incorporate Leafy Greens**:

   o **Daily Intake**: Aim to include a variety of leafy greens in your daily diet. Spinach, kale, collard greens, and Swiss chard are excellent options.

   o **Meal Ideas**: Add spinach to smoothies, sauté kale with garlic and olive oil as a side dish, use collard greens as a wrap for sandwiches, and mix Swiss chard into soups and stews.

1. **Include Beets**:

   o **Versatile Use**: Beets can be enjoyed in many forms, including raw, roasted, steamed, or juiced. They can also be added to salads, soups, and smoothies.

   o **Meal Ideas**: Roast beets with a drizzle of olive oil and balsamic vinegar, blend beets into a smoothie with berries and spinach, or slice raw beets thinly for a crunchy salad topping.

1. **Add Bananas**:

   o **Convenient Snack**: Bananas are a convenient and portable snack that can be enjoyed on their own or added to various dishes.

   o **Meal Ideas**: Slice bananas onto oatmeal or yogurt, blend into smoothies, or enjoy as a natural sweetener in baked goods.

1. **Incorporate Seeds**:

- **Easy Addition**: Seeds can be easily added to a variety of dishes to boost their nutritional content.
- **Meal Ideas**: Sprinkle chia seeds onto yogurt or oatmeal, add flaxseeds to smoothies or baked goods, and enjoy pumpkin seeds as a crunchy salad topping or snack.

Sample Meal Plan for Blood Pressure Management

Breakfast:

- **Green Smoothie**: Blend spinach, banana, chia seeds, and almond milk for a nutrient-packed smoothie rich in potassium and fiber.
- **Oatmeal with Flaxseeds**: Top a bowl of oatmeal with flaxseeds, fresh berries, and a drizzle of honey.

Lunch:

- **Beet Salad**: Toss roasted beets with arugula, goat cheese, walnuts, and a balsamic vinaigrette.
- **Quinoa and Kale Bowl**: Combine cooked quinoa with sautéed kale, chickpeas, cherry tomatoes, and avocado, dressed with lemon-tahini sauce.

Snack:

- **Banana and Nut Butter**: Enjoy a banana with a spoonful of almond or peanut butter for a balanced snack.
- **Pumpkin Seeds**: Snack on a handful of roasted pumpkin seeds.

Dinner:

- **Stir-Fried Vegetables**: Stir-fry a mix of leafy greens (such as bok choy and spinach), bell peppers, and tofu with garlic, ginger, and a splash of low-sodium soy sauce.

- **Roasted Beet and Sweet Potato**: Serve roasted beets and sweet potatoes as a side dish, seasoned with olive oil, rosemary, and black pepper.

Dessert:

- **Chia Seed Pudding**: Mix chia seeds with almond milk and a touch of vanilla extract. Let it sit overnight and top with fresh fruit before serving.

Spiritual and Community Support

1. **Faith and Prayer**:

   o   Incorporating faith and prayer into daily life can provide emotional and spiritual support, reducing stress, which is a significant factor in hypertension. Regular prayer and meditation can cultivate a sense of peace and well-being, aiding in blood pressure management.

1. **Community Engagement**:

   o   Engaging with a faith community can offer encouragement and accountability in making healthy lifestyle choices. Community activities such as communal meals, cooking classes, and walking clubs can promote a plant-based diet and physical activity, contributing to better blood pressure control.

1. **Education and Advocacy**:

   o   Churches and faith-based organizations can play a crucial role in educating members about the importance of a healthy diet for managing blood pressure. Hosting workshops, seminars, and health fairs can disseminate valuable information and resources.

The inclusion of leafy greens, beets, bananas, and seeds in the diet aligns with both biblical wisdom and modern scientific understanding. These potassium-rich foods are essential for managing blood pressure and promoting overall cardiovascular health.

By incorporating these foods into your daily diet, you can create balanced, satisfying meals that nourish your body and support your health. Embracing the principles of natural, whole foods as taught in the Bible helps you maintain a healthy relationship with food and honors the divine wisdom of caring for your body. As a Christian preacher and seasoned nutritionist, I encourage you to reflect on the timeless teachings of Scripture and apply them to your dietary choices. By doing so, you can achieve better health, prevent and manage hypertension, and enjoy the abundant life that

Detailed Analysis and Benefits of Each Food

Leafy Greens

Spinach, Kale, Collard Greens, Swiss Chard
   Nutritional Powerhouses:
- Leafy greens are low in calories but high in vitamins, minerals, and fiber. They are particularly rich in vitamin K, which helps in blood clotting and bone health, and vitamin A, which is essential for vision and immune function.
- **Potassium Content**: Leafy greens are excellent sources of potassium, which helps to counteract the effects of sodium in the body, thus reducing blood pressure. For instance, one cup of cooked spinach contains about 839 mg of potassium.

   Impact on Blood Pressure:
- **Scientific Evidence**: Studies have shown that a higher intake of leafy greens is associated with a reduced risk of hypertension. The high

potassium content helps relax blood vessels and promotes sodium excretion through urine.

- **Antioxidant Properties**: Leafy greens are rich in antioxidants, such as beta-carotene and lutein, which reduce oxidative stress and inflammation, contributing to lower blood pressure.

Practical Tips:

- **Smoothies**: Incorporate spinach or kale into smoothies for a nutrient boost without compromising taste.
- **Salads**: Use a mix of leafy greens as a base for salads, adding a variety of colorful vegetables, nuts, and seeds for a balanced meal.
- **Cooking**: Sauté or steam greens as a side dish, or add them to soups and stews for added nutrition.

Beets

Nutrient-Rich Root Vegetables

Nutritional Profile:

- Beets are rich in essential nutrients, including fiber, folate, vitamin C, and potassium. They also contain pigments called betalains, which have anti-inflammatory and antioxidant properties.
- **Potassium Content**: A cup of beet juice can contain around 500 mg of potassium, which is beneficial for blood pressure control.

Impact on Blood Pressure:

- **Dietary Nitrates**: Beets are high in dietary nitrates, which the body converts into nitric oxide. Nitric oxide helps relax and widen blood vessels, improving blood flow and reducing blood pressure.
- **Scientific Evidence**: Research has shown that consuming beet juice can lower systolic and diastolic blood pressure. A study in the journal Hypertension found that participants who drank beet juice experienced significant reductions in blood pressure.

Practical Tips:

- **Juicing**: Make fresh beet juice or include beets in vegetable juice blends.
- **Roasting**: Roast beets with olive oil and herbs for a delicious side dish.
- **Salads**: Add roasted or raw beets to salads for a sweet, earthy flavor and a nutritional boost.

Bananas

Convenient and Nutritious Fruits

Nutritional Profile:

- Bananas are well-known for their high potassium content, with a medium-sized banana providing approximately 400-450 mg of potassium. They are also a good source of vitamin C, vitamin B6, and dietary fiber.
- **Natural Energy Source**: Bananas provide a quick source of energy due to their natural sugars and high fiber content, which helps regulate blood sugar levels.

Impact on Blood Pressure:

- **Potassium's Role**: Potassium helps balance sodium levels in the body, reducing water retention and lowering blood pressure. This mineral is essential for maintaining healthy heart function and controlling blood pressure.
- **Scientific Evidence**: Studies have consistently shown that potassium-rich diets are associated with lower blood pressure and reduced risk of stroke. The American Heart Association recommends increasing potassium intake to help manage blood pressure.

Practical Tips:

- **Snacking**: Bananas make an easy and portable snack.

- **Smoothies**: Blend bananas into smoothies for natural sweetness and added nutrients.
- **Baking**: Use mashed bananas as a natural sweetener in baking, reducing the need for added sugars.

Seeds

Flaxseeds, Chia Seeds, Pumpkin Seeds
Nutritional Powerhouses:
- Seeds are rich in omega-3 fatty acids, protein, fiber, and essential minerals such as magnesium, zinc, and potassium. They provide a concentrated source of nutrition that supports heart health and overall well-being.
- **Potassium Content**: Seeds like pumpkin seeds are particularly high in potassium, with one cup of pumpkin seeds providing about 588 mg of potassium.

Impact on Blood Pressure:
- **Omega-3 Fatty Acids**: Seeds are excellent sources of alpha-linolenic acid (ALA), a type of omega-3 fatty acid that has anti-inflammatory effects and can help lower blood pressure.
- **Magnesium and Zinc**: These minerals support cardiovascular health by helping to regulate blood pressure and prevent the buildup of plaque in arteries.
- **Scientific Evidence**: Research has shown that the regular consumption of seeds can improve lipid profiles, reduce blood pressure, and decrease the risk of cardiovascular diseases.

Practical Tips:
- **Toppings**: Sprinkle seeds on top of yogurt, oatmeal, or salads for added crunch and nutrition.

- **Smoothies**: Blend chia or flaxseeds into smoothies for a nutrient boost.
- **Baking**: Incorporate seeds into baked goods such as bread, muffins, and granola bars.

Spiritual and Community Support

1. **Faith and Prayer**:

   o Incorporating faith and prayer into daily life can provide emotional and spiritual support, reducing stress, which is a significant factor in hypertension. Regular prayer and meditation can cultivate a sense of peace and well-being, aiding in blood pressure management.

1. **Community Engagement**:

   o Engaging with a faith community can offer encouragement and accountability in making healthy lifestyle choices. Community activities such as communal meals, cooking classes, and walking clubs can promote a plant-based diet and physical activity, contributing to better blood pressure control.

1. **Education and Advocacy**:

   o Churches and faith-based organizations can play a crucial role in educating members about the importance of a healthy diet for managing blood pressure. Hosting workshops, seminars, and health fairs can disseminate valuable information and resources.

Integrating Faith and Nutrition for Holistic Health

Combining spiritual practices with healthy eating habits can lead to holistic well-being. Here are some practical steps to integrate faith and nutrition into your lifestyle:

1. **Start with Prayer**:

    o   Begin each meal with a prayer of gratitude, acknowledging God's provision and asking for His blessing on the food. This practice fosters a mindful approach to eating and reinforces the connection between faith and health.

1. **Scripture Study and Reflection**:

    o   Study biblical passages that highlight the importance of caring for the body, such as 1 Corinthians 6:19-20 and Proverbs 3:7-8. Reflect on how these teachings can guide your dietary choices and overall lifestyle.

1. **Community Support**:

    o   Participate in or organize church-based health initiatives, such as cooking classes that focus on preparing healthy, plant-based meals or group exercise sessions that promote physical activity and fellowship.

1. **Fasting and Spiritual Renewal**:

    o   Incorporate periodic fasting as a spiritual discipline that also offers physical health benefits. Use fasting periods to pray, reflect, and draw closer to God, while giving your body a break from constant digestion and processing of food.

The inclusion of leafy greens, beets, bananas, and seeds in the diet aligns with both biblical wisdom and modern scientific understanding. These potassium-rich foods are essential for managing blood pressure and promoting overall cardiovascular health.

By incorporating these foods into your daily diet, you can create balanced, satisfying meals that nourish your body and support your health. Embracing the principles of natural, whole foods as taught in the Bible helps you maintain a healthy relationship with food and honors the divine wisdom of caring for your body.

Chapter 9: Foods to Avoid

High-Sodium Foods and Processed Meats

In the journey toward better health and well-being, understanding the foods to avoid is just as crucial as knowing what to include in our diets. High-sodium foods and processed meats pose significant risks to heart health, and their prevalence in modern diets has made it imperative to address these concerns from both a biblical and scientific perspective.

Biblical Perspective on Diet and Health

The Bible, with its timeless wisdom, offers guidance on moderation, purity, and the consumption of wholesome foods. Although specific references to sodium and processed meats are not found in Scripture, the underlying principles of moderation, purity, and health can be applied to our understanding of these modern dietary concerns.

1. **Moderation and Self-Control**:

- **Proverbs 25:16**: "If you find honey, eat just enough—too much of it, and you will vomit."
- This proverb highlights the importance of moderation in all things. While honey represents natural sweetness, the principle can be extended to all aspects of diet, including sodium intake. Consuming excessive amounts of anything, including salt, can lead to detrimental health effects.

1. **Purity and Wholesomeness**:

- **Daniel 1:8**: "But Daniel resolved not to defile himself with the royal food and wine, and he asked the chief official for permission not to defile himself this way."
- Daniel's refusal to consume the king's rich, processed foods in favor of a simple, wholesome diet of vegetables and water demonstrates a commitment to purity and health. This principle encourages us to choose natural, unprocessed foods over those laden with unhealthy additives.

1. **The Body as a Temple**:

- **1 Corinthians 6:19-20**: "Do you not know that your bodies are temples of the Holy Spirit, who is in you, whom you have received from God? You are not your own; you were bought at a price. Therefore honor God with your bodies."
- This passage underscores the responsibility to care for our bodies. Avoiding harmful substances, such as excessive sodium and processed meats, is part of honoring our bodies as temples of the Holy Spirit.

The Impact of Sodium on Heart Health

Sodium is an essential mineral that the body needs to function properly. It helps maintain fluid balance, supports nerve function, and influences muscle contraction. However, excessive sodium intake can have severe consequences on heart health.

1. **Blood Pressure and Hypertension**:

- High sodium intake is directly linked to elevated blood pressure, a primary risk factor for heart disease and stroke. Sodium causes the body to retain water, increasing the volume of blood and, consequently, the pressure on blood vessel walls.
- **Scientific Evidence**: The American Heart Association states that reducing sodium intake can significantly lower blood pressure and reduce the risk of cardiovascular diseases.

1. **Heart Disease and Stroke**:

- Excessive sodium consumption contributes to the development of heart disease and stroke. It can lead to hypertensive heart disease, heart failure, and other cardiovascular conditions.
- **Scientific Evidence**: A study published in the New England Journal of Medicine found that high sodium intake is associated with an increased risk of heart disease and stroke. Reducing sodium intake to recommended levels could prevent numerous cases of heart disease.

1. **Kidney Function**:

- The kidneys play a crucial role in regulating sodium levels in the body. High sodium intake puts extra strain on the kidneys, leading to potential kidney damage and increased risk of kidney disease.
- **Scientific Evidence**: Research in the journal Hypertension indicates that reducing sodium intake can improve kidney function and reduce the risk of kidney disease, which is often associated with high blood pressure.

Processed Meats and Their Health Risks

Processed meats, such as bacon, sausages, hot dogs, and deli meats, are meats that have been preserved by smoking, curing, salting, or adding chemical preservatives. These meats pose significant health risks, particularly in relation to heart health.

1. **High Sodium Content**:

- Processed meats are typically high in sodium, which, as discussed, can lead to hypertension and cardiovascular diseases.
- **Example**: A single serving of processed meat can contain more than half of the recommended daily sodium intake, contributing significantly to excessive sodium consumption.

1. **Saturated Fats and Trans Fats**:

- Processed meats often contain high levels of saturated fats and trans fats, which can raise LDL (bad) cholesterol levels and lower HDL (good) cholesterol levels, increasing the risk of heart disease.
- **Scientific Evidence**: Studies published in the American Journal of Clinical Nutrition have shown a strong link between the consumption of processed meats and increased risk of coronary artery disease.

1. **Carcinogenic Compounds**:

- Processed meats contain nitrites and nitrates, preservatives that can form carcinogenic compounds known as nitrosamines during cooking or digestion. These compounds have been linked to an increased risk of certain cancers, including colorectal cancer.
- **Scientific Evidence**: The World Health Organization's International Agency for Research on Cancer (IARC) has classified

processed meats as Group 1 carcinogens, meaning there is sufficient evidence of their carcinogenicity in humans.

Modern Relevance: The Dangers of Processed Foods and Sugary Drinks

In today's fast-paced world, processed foods and sugary drinks have become staples in many diets. Understanding their dangers and learning to avoid them is crucial for maintaining good health.

1. **Processed Foods**:

   o   Processed foods are often high in added sugars, unhealthy fats, and sodium. They are typically low in essential nutrients such as fiber, vitamins, and minerals. Consuming these foods regularly can lead to various health issues.

   o   **Examples**: Snack cakes, cookies, breakfast cereals, and fast food items often contain high-fructose corn syrup, trans fats, and artificial additives.

1. **Sugary Drinks**:

   o   Sugary drinks, including sodas, fruit juices, and energy drinks, are significant sources of added sugars in the diet. They provide empty calories without any nutritional benefits and contribute to the risk of obesity, diabetes, and other chronic diseases.

   o   **Examples**: Regular soda, sweetened iced tea, lemonade, and many commercially available fruit juices and sports drinks are loaded with sugars.

Health Impacts:

- **Weight Gain and Obesity**: Sugary drinks contribute significantly to weight gain due to their high sugar content and low satiety value. This can lead to an increased risk of obesity-related diseases.

- **Type 2 Diabetes**: The rapid absorption of sugars from sugary drinks causes spikes in blood sugar and insulin levels, increasing the risk of insulin resistance and type 2 diabetes.
- **Dental Problems**: Sugary drinks are a major cause of tooth decay and cavities. The high sugar content provides food for bacteria in the mouth, leading to acid production and tooth enamel erosion.

Practical Steps to Reduce Sodium and Avoid Processed Meats

1. **Read Food Labels**:

    - **Identify Sodium Content**: Check food labels for sodium content and choose products with lower sodium levels. Be aware of hidden sources of sodium in foods such as bread, canned vegetables, and sauces.
    - **Choose Whole Foods**: Opt for whole, unprocessed foods whenever possible. Fresh fruits, vegetables, whole grains, and lean proteins should be the foundation of your diet.

1. **Cook at Home**:

    - **Control Ingredients**: Cooking at home allows you to control the ingredients in your meals, reducing the likelihood of consuming added sodium and unhealthy fats.
    - **Healthy Recipes**: Experiment with healthy recipes that use fresh, natural ingredients. This not only improves nutrition but also enhances the flavor and enjoyment of meals.

1. **Limit Processed Meats**:

- **Healthier Alternatives**: Choose lean cuts of fresh meat, poultry, and fish instead of processed meats. Consider plant-based protein sources such as beans, lentils, and tofu.
- **Preparation Methods**: Grill, bake, or steam meats instead of frying or using high-sodium marinades and sauces.

1. **Use Herbs and Spices**:

- **Flavor Without Sodium**: Use herbs, spices, garlic, lemon juice, and vinegar to add flavor to your meals without adding sodium. Fresh herbs like basil, cilantro, and parsley can enhance the taste of dishes naturally.
- **Homemade Seasonings**: Create your own seasoning blends using herbs and spices to reduce reliance on pre-packaged seasoning mixes that may contain high sodium levels.

1. **Hydrate Wisely**:

- **Water First**: Make water your primary beverage. Add slices of fruit or herbs for flavor if needed. Herbal teas and infused water are also good options.
- **Limit Sugary Drinks**: Avoid sugary drinks and opt for healthier alternatives. If you crave something sweet, try making a smoothie with fresh fruits and a source of protein, such as Greek yogurt or a handful of nuts.

1. **Plan and Prepare**:

- **Meal Prep**: Plan and prepare meals ahead of time to ensure you have healthy options available. This reduces the temptation to choose processed foods or sugary snacks when you are hungry.
- **Balanced Meals**: Ensure each meal includes a balance of macronutrients: proteins, fats, and carbohydrates. This helps maintain energy levels and prevents blood sugar spikes.

Sample Meal Plan to Avoid High-Sodium Foods and Processed Meats

Breakfast:

- **Oatmeal with Fresh Fruit**: Top a bowl of oatmeal with fresh berries, sliced banana, and a sprinkle of flaxseeds. Sweeten with a touch of honey or maple syrup if desired.
- **Green Smoothie**: Blend spinach, banana, chia seeds, and almond milk for a nutrient-packed smoothie.

Lunch:

- **Quinoa Salad**: Combine cooked quinoa with diced cucumbers, cherry tomatoes, red onion, and parsley. Dress with lemon juice and olive oil.
- **Lentil Soup**: Make a hearty lentil soup with carrots, celery, onions, and tomatoes. Season with garlic, thyme, and bay leaves.

Snack:

- **Fresh Fruit and Nuts**: Enjoy an apple with a handful of almonds or a pear with a small serving of walnuts.
- **Veggie Sticks and Hummus**: Snack on sliced bell peppers, carrots, and cucumbers dipped in hummus.

Dinner:

- **Grilled Salmon**: Grill a salmon fillet seasoned with herbs and lemon. Serve with a side of steamed broccoli and brown rice.
- **Vegetable Stir-Fry**: Stir-fry a mix of colorful vegetables such as bell peppers, snap peas, and mushrooms with tofu or chicken breast. Season with low-sodium soy sauce, ginger, and garlic.

Dessert:

- **Fruit Salad**: Combine a variety of fresh fruits such as berries, melon, and kiwi for a refreshing dessert. Add a sprinkle of mint for extra flavor.

Integrating Faith and Nutrition for Holistic Health

Combining spiritual practices with healthy eating habits can lead to holistic well-being. Here are some practical steps to integrate faith and nutrition into your lifestyle:

1. **Start with Prayer**:

   - Begin each meal with a prayer of gratitude, acknowledging God's provision and asking for His blessing on the food. This practice fosters a mindful approach to eating and reinforces the connection between faith and health.

1. **Scripture Study and Reflection**:

   - Study biblical passages that highlight the importance of caring for the body, such as 1 Corinthians 6:19-20 and Proverbs 3:7-8. Reflect on how these teachings can guide your dietary choices and overall lifestyle.

1. **Community Support**:

   - Participate in or organize church-based health initiatives, such as cooking classes that focus on preparing healthy, plant-based meals or group exercise sessions that promote physical activity and fellowship.

1. **Fasting and Spiritual Renewal**:

   - Incorporate periodic fasting as a spiritual discipline that also offers physical health benefits. Use fasting periods to pray, reflect, and draw closer to God, while giving your body a break from constant digestion and processing of food.

Avoiding high-sodium foods and processed meats is crucial for maintaining heart health and overall well-being. By understanding the biblical principles of moderation, purity, and honoring our bodies, we can make informed dietary choices that support our health and reflect our faith.

The dangers of excessive sodium intake and processed meats are well-documented by scientific research. By reducing consumption of these harmful foods and opting for fresh, natural alternatives, we can significantly reduce the risk of hypertension, heart disease, and other chronic conditions.

As a Christian preacher and seasoned nutritionist, I encourage you to reflect on the timeless teachings of Scripture and apply them to your dietary choices. By doing so, you can achieve better health, prevent and manage chronic diseases, and enjoy the abundant life that God intends for you. Let us seek God's guidance in our dietary practices and trust in His provision for our health and vitality.

Part 4: Biblical Diet for Cholesterol

Chapter 10: Cholesterol in Biblical Context

Cholesterol is a waxy, fat-like substance found in all the cells of the body. While it is essential for the formation of cell membranes, hormones, and vitamin D, high levels of cholesterol in the blood can lead to serious health problems, including heart disease. In this chapter, we will explore the biblical perspective on diet, particularly the importance of fruits and vegetables, and how these principles can help manage cholesterol levels and improve heart health.

Explanation of Cholesterol and Heart Health

Cholesterol travels through the bloodstream in small packages called lipoproteins, which are made of fat (lipid) on the inside and proteins on the outside. There are two main types of lipoproteins that carry cholesterol throughout the body:

1. **Low-Density Lipoprotein (LDL):**

- Often referred to as "bad" cholesterol, LDL carries cholesterol from the liver to the cells. High levels of LDL cholesterol can lead to a buildup of cholesterol in the arteries, forming plaques that narrow and harden the arteries. This condition, known as atherosclerosis, can restrict blood flow and increase the risk of heart attacks and strokes.

1. **High-Density Lipoprotein (HDL):**

- Known as "good" cholesterol, HDL carries cholesterol from other parts of the body back to the liver, where it is removed from the body. High levels of HDL cholesterol are associated with a lower risk of heart disease because HDL helps clear cholesterol from the bloodstream.

Maintaining a healthy balance between LDL and HDL cholesterol is crucial for cardiovascular health. Diet plays a significant role in managing cholesterol levels, and incorporating biblical principles can provide a foundation for making heart-healthy dietary choices.

Ezekiel 47:12 – "Their fruit will serve for food and their leaves for healing."

This verse from Ezekiel highlights the importance of fruits and vegetables, emphasizing their role in providing nourishment and healing. The biblical emphasis on natural, plant-based foods aligns with modern nutritional science, which supports the consumption of fruits and vegetables for maintaining healthy cholesterol levels and promoting overall heart health.

Importance of Fruits and Vegetables

Fruits and vegetables are rich in essential nutrients, fiber, antioxidants, and phytochemicals that contribute to heart health and help manage cholesterol levels. Here are some key benefits of including a variety of fruits and vegetables in your diet:

1. **High in Soluble Fiber**:

- Soluble fiber, found in fruits, vegetables, and whole grains, helps lower LDL cholesterol levels by binding to cholesterol in the digestive system and removing it from the body. Foods high in soluble fiber include apples, oranges, pears, berries, carrots, broccoli, and Brussels sprouts.

1. **Rich in Antioxidants**:

- Antioxidants such as vitamins C and E, found in many fruits and vegetables, protect the body from oxidative stress and inflammation, which are contributing factors to atherosclerosis and heart disease. Berries, citrus fruits, and leafy greens are particularly high in antioxidants.

1. **Phytochemicals and Plant Sterols**:

- Phytochemicals are naturally occurring compounds in plants that have various health benefits, including lowering cholesterol levels and reducing the risk of heart disease. Plant sterols, found in fruits, vegetables, nuts, and seeds, help block the absorption of cholesterol in the intestines.

1. **Low in Saturated Fat and Calories**:

- Fruits and vegetables are naturally low in saturated fat and calories, making them ideal for maintaining a healthy weight and reducing the risk of high cholesterol and heart disease. Incorporating these foods into your diet can help manage weight and improve overall health.

Practical Application of a Biblical Diet for Cholesterol Management

Implementing a biblical diet rich in fruits and vegetables can be both simple and effective. Here are practical steps and dietary strategies to help manage cholesterol levels and promote heart health.

1. **Increase Fruit and Vegetable Intake**:

- Aim to fill half your plate with fruits and vegetables at each meal. Include a wide range of colors and types to ensure a diverse intake of nutrients.
- **Meal Ideas**: Add berries to your morning oatmeal, include a side salad with lunch, and incorporate roasted vegetables into your dinner.

1. **Choose Whole Fruits and Vegetables**:

- Opt for whole fruits and vegetables rather than juices or processed versions to maximize fiber intake and reduce added sugars.
- **Examples**: Eat an apple instead of drinking apple juice, snack on carrot sticks instead of processed veggie chips.

1. **Incorporate Leafy Greens**:

- Leafy greens such as spinach, kale, and Swiss chard are particularly high in nutrients and fiber. Add them to salads, smoothies, and soups.
- **Meal Ideas**: Make a green smoothie with spinach, banana, and almond milk; add kale to a hearty vegetable soup; use Swiss chard as a wrap for lean proteins.

1. **Include Nuts and Seeds**:

  o   Nuts and seeds are rich in healthy fats, fiber, and plant sterols. They can be a great addition to meals or snacks.

  o   **Examples**: Sprinkle chia seeds on yogurt, add walnuts to a salad, or enjoy a handful of almonds as a snack.

1. **Use Healthy Fats**:

  o   Replace saturated fats with healthy fats from plant sources, such as olive oil, avocados, and nuts. These fats can help improve cholesterol levels and support heart health.

  o   **Cooking Tips**: Use olive oil for sautéing vegetables, add avocado slices to sandwiches and salads, and use nut butters as a spread or dip.

Sample Meal Plan for Cholesterol Management

Breakfast:

- **Berry Oatmeal**: Cook oatmeal with almond milk and top with fresh berries, a sprinkle of chia seeds, and a drizzle of honey.
- **Green Smoothie**: Blend spinach, banana, kiwi, and flaxseeds with water or almond milk for a nutrient-rich smoothie.

Lunch:

- **Quinoa Salad**: Combine cooked quinoa with diced cucumbers, cherry tomatoes, red onion, and parsley. Dress with lemon juice and olive oil.
- **Vegetable Wrap**: Use a large Swiss chard leaf as a wrap and fill with hummus, sliced bell peppers, cucumbers, and shredded carrots.

Snack:

- **Fruit and Nut Mix**: Enjoy a mix of dried fruits (such as apricots and raisins) and nuts (such as almonds and walnuts).

- **Veggie Sticks and Guacamole**: Snack on sliced bell peppers, carrots, and celery with a side of guacamole.

Dinner:

- **Grilled Salmon**: Grill a salmon fillet seasoned with herbs and lemon. Serve with a side of steamed broccoli and a sweet potato.
- **Stuffed Bell Peppers**: Fill bell peppers with a mixture of brown rice, black beans, corn, and diced tomatoes. Top with avocado slices and cilantro.

Dessert:

- **Fruit Salad**: Combine a variety of fresh fruits such as berries, melon, and kiwi for a refreshing dessert. Add a sprinkle of mint for extra flavor.

Integrating Faith and Nutrition for Holistic Health

Combining spiritual practices with healthy eating habits can lead to holistic well-being. Here are some practical steps to integrate faith and nutrition into your lifestyle:

1. **Start with Prayer**:

   - Begin each meal with a prayer of gratitude, acknowledging God's provision and asking for His blessing on the food. This practice fosters a mindful approach to eating and reinforces the connection between faith and health.

1. **Scripture Study and Reflection**:

   - Study biblical passages that highlight the importance of caring for the body, such as 1 Corinthians 6:19-20 and Proverbs 3:7-8. Reflect on how these teachings can guide your dietary choices and overall lifestyle.

1. **Community Support**:

- Participate in or organize church-based health initiatives, such as cooking classes that focus on preparing healthy, plant-based meals or group exercise sessions that promote physical activity and fellowship.

1. **Fasting and Spiritual Renewal:**

   - Incorporate periodic fasting as a spiritual discipline that also offers physical health benefits. Use fasting periods to pray, reflect, and draw closer to God, while giving your body a break from constant digestion and processing of food.

The Role of Faith and Community in Health

1. **Spiritual Support:**

   - Incorporating faith and prayer into daily life can provide emotional and spiritual support, reducing stress, which is a significant factor in heart health. Regular prayer and meditation can help cultivate a sense of peace and well-being.

1. **Community Engagement:**

   - Engaging with a faith community can offer encouragement and accountability in making healthy lifestyle choices. Community activities such as communal meals, cooking classes, and walking clubs can promote a plant-based diet and physical activity.

1. **Education and Advocacy:**

   - Churches and faith-based organizations can play a crucial role in educating members about the importance of a healthy diet for managing cholesterol. Hosting workshops, seminars, and health fairs can disseminate valuable information and resources.

The inclusion of fruits and vegetables in the diet aligns with both biblical wisdom and modern scientific understanding. These foods are essential for managing cholesterol levels and promoting overall cardiovascular health.

By incorporating a variety of fruits and vegetables into your daily diet, you can create balanced, satisfying meals that nourish your body and support your health. Embracing the principles of natural, whole foods as taught in the Bible helps you maintain a healthy relationship with food and honors the divine wisdom of caring for your body.

As a Christian preacher and seasoned nutritionist, I encourage you to reflect on the timeless teachings of Scripture and apply them to your dietary choices. By doing so, you can achieve better health, prevent and manage high cholesterol, and enjoy the abundant life that God intends for you. Let us seek God's guidance in our dietary practices and trust in His provision for our health and vitality.

Chapter 11: Foods to Include

Oats, Barley, Beans, and Fatty Fish

The Bible provides timeless guidance on the importance of a healthy diet, emphasizing natural and wholesome foods. Incorporating oats, barley, beans, and fatty fish into our diets aligns with both biblical principles and modern nutritional science. These foods are rich in soluble fiber and omega-3 fatty acids, which play crucial roles in managing cholesterol levels and promoting overall heart health. In this chapter, we will explore the biblical basis for these foods, their health benefits, and their modern relevance.

Biblical Perspective on Oats, Barley, Beans, and Fatty Fish

The consumption of natural, nutrient-dense foods is deeply rooted in biblical teachings. While oats and fatty fish are not explicitly mentioned in the Bible, the principles of consuming wholesome, God-given foods can be applied to these items. Barley and beans, however, are directly referenced in Scripture, highlighting their significance.

1. **Barley**:

- **Ezekiel 4:9**: "Take also unto thee wheat, and barley, and beans, and lentils, and millet, and spelt, and put them in one vessel, and make thee bread thereof."
- Barley is mentioned as a staple grain in the Bible, valued for its nutritional content and used in bread-making. It symbolizes sustenance and health.

1. **Beans**:

- **2 Samuel 17:28-29**: "Brought beds, and basins, and earthen vessels, and wheat, and barley, and flour, and parched corn, and beans, and lentils, and parched pulse, And honey, and butter, and sheep, and cheese of kine, for David, and for the people that were with him, to eat."
- Beans are highlighted as an important food source, providing essential nutrients and protein. They were part of the diet that sustained King David and his people.

1. **Oats**:

- While oats are not specifically mentioned in the Bible, they are a whole grain similar to wheat and barley. The biblical emphasis on grains as a source of nourishment extends to oats, which offer significant health benefits.

1. **Fatty Fish**:

- **John 21:9-13**: "When they landed, they saw a fire of burning coals there with fish on it, and some bread. Jesus said to them, 'Bring some of the fish you have just caught.'"
- Fish is a recurring element in biblical narratives, symbolizing sustenance and provision. While fatty fish like salmon and mackerel are not specified, the inclusion of fish in the diet aligns with biblical principles of consuming natural, health-promoting foods.

Health Benefits of Oats, Barley, Beans, and Fatty Fish

1. **Oats**:

- **Nutrient-Dense**: Oats are rich in vitamins, minerals, antioxidants, and fiber. They provide essential nutrients such as manganese, phosphorus, magnesium, copper, iron, zinc, folate, and vitamin B1.
- **Soluble Fiber**: Oats are an excellent source of soluble fiber, particularly beta-glucan, which helps lower LDL cholesterol levels by forming a gel-like substance in the gut that binds to cholesterol-rich bile acids and removes them from the body.
- **Scientific Evidence**: Numerous studies, including those published in the American Journal of Clinical Nutrition, have shown that consuming oats can reduce LDL cholesterol levels and improve heart health.

1. **Barley**:

- **Nutrient-Rich**: Barley is high in vitamins, minerals, and fiber. It contains significant amounts of selenium, manganese, magnesium, copper, and vitamin B1.
- **Soluble Fiber**: Like oats, barley is rich in beta-glucan, a soluble fiber that helps lower cholesterol levels by binding to bile acids and reducing their reabsorption.

- **Scientific Evidence**: Research published in the Journal of Nutrition indicates that barley consumption can significantly reduce total and LDL cholesterol levels, improving cardiovascular health.

1. **Beans**:

- **High in Protein and Fiber**: Beans are an excellent source of plant-based protein and dietary fiber. They provide essential nutrients such as folate, iron, magnesium, and potassium.
- **Soluble Fiber**: Beans contain soluble fiber that helps lower cholesterol levels by binding to bile acids and promoting their excretion. The fiber also supports healthy digestion and prevents constipation.
- **Scientific Evidence**: Studies, including those in the Archives of Internal Medicine, have shown that regular consumption of beans can lower LDL cholesterol and improve overall heart health.

1. **Fatty Fish**:

- **Rich in Omega-3 Fatty Acids**: Fatty fish such as salmon, mackerel, sardines, and trout are rich in omega-3 fatty acids, which have anti-inflammatory properties and support heart health. Omega-3s help lower triglycerides, reduce blood pressure, and prevent plaque formation in arteries.
- **Protein and Nutrients**: Fatty fish are also high in high-quality protein and essential nutrients such as vitamin D, selenium, and iodine.
- **Scientific Evidence**: Numerous studies, including those published in the Journal of the American Medical Association, have shown that regular consumption of fatty fish reduces the risk of heart disease and improves overall cardiovascular health.

Modern Relevance: Soluble Fiber and Omega-3 Fatty Acids for Cholesterol Management

Soluble fiber and omega-3 fatty acids are essential for managing cholesterol levels and promoting heart health. Here is how they work and why they are important:

1. **Soluble Fiber**:

  o **Mechanism**: Soluble fiber forms a gel-like substance in the gut that binds to cholesterol-rich bile acids, which are then excreted from the body. This process reduces the amount of cholesterol absorbed into the bloodstream.

  o **Sources**: Foods rich in soluble fiber include oats, barley, beans, apples, pears, and carrots.

  o **Benefits**: Regular consumption of soluble fiber helps lower LDL cholesterol levels, reduces the risk of heart disease, and promotes healthy digestion.

1. **Omega-3 Fatty Acids**:

  o **Mechanism**: Omega-3 fatty acids reduce inflammation, lower triglycerides, decrease blood pressure, and prevent the formation of plaques in the arteries. They also help maintain the stability of the heart's electrical activity, reducing the risk of arrhythmias.

  o **Sources**: Foods rich in omega-3 fatty acids include fatty fish (salmon, mackerel, sardines), flaxseeds, chia seeds, walnuts, and algae.

  o **Benefits**: Regular consumption of omega-3 fatty acids supports cardiovascular health, improves cholesterol levels, and reduces the risk of heart disease and stroke.

Practical Steps to Incorporate Oats, Barley, Beans, and Fatty Fish into the Diet

1. **Oats**:

- **Breakfast**: Start your day with a bowl of oatmeal topped with fresh berries, nuts, and a drizzle of honey.
- **Baking**: Use oats in baking recipes such as muffins, cookies, and bread for added fiber and nutrients.
- **Smoothies**: Add a handful of oats to smoothies for a creamy texture and additional fiber.

1. **Barley**:

- **Soups and Stews**: Add barley to soups and stews for a hearty and nutritious meal.
- **Salads**: Use cooked barley as a base for salads, combined with vegetables, beans, and a light vinaigrette.
- **Side Dishes**: Serve barley as a side dish instead of rice or pasta, flavored with herbs and olive oil.

1. **Beans**:

- **Salads**: Add beans to salads for extra protein and fiber. Black beans, chickpeas, and kidney beans are great options.
- **Soups and Stews**: Use beans in soups and stews to create filling and nutritious meals.
- **Dips and Spreads**: Make bean dips and spreads, such as hummus or black bean dip, for healthy snacks and appetizers.

1. **Fatty Fish**:

- **Grilled or Baked**: Grill or bake fatty fish with herbs and lemon for a flavorful and heart-healthy meal.

- **Salads and Sandwiches**: Add flaked salmon or mackerel to salads and sandwiches for a boost of omega-3 fatty acids.
- **Tacos**: Make fish tacos using grilled or baked fish, topped with fresh vegetables and a squeeze of lime.

Sample Meal Plan for Cholesterol Management

Breakfast:

- **Berry Oatmeal**: Cook oatmeal with almond milk and top with fresh berries, a sprinkle of chia seeds, and a drizzle of honey.
- **Green Smoothie**: Blend spinach, banana, oats, and flaxseeds with water or almond milk for a nutrient-rich smoothie.

Lunch:

- **Barley Salad**: Combine cooked barley with diced cucumbers, cherry tomatoes, red onion, and parsley. Dress with lemon juice and olive oil.
- **Bean and Veggie Wrap**: Use a whole grain wrap filled with black beans, avocado, shredded lettuce, and salsa.

Snack:

- **Fruit and Nut Mix**: Enjoy a mix of dried fruits (such as apricots and raisins) and nuts (such as almonds and walnuts).
- **Veggie Sticks and Hummus**: Snack on sliced bell peppers, carrots, and celery with a side of hummus.

Dinner:

- **Grilled Salmon**: Grill a salmon fillet seasoned with herbs and lemon. Serve with a side of steamed broccoli and quinoa.
- **Bean Chili**: Make a hearty bean chili with kidney beans, black beans, tomatoes, bell peppers, and spices. Serve with a slice of whole grain bread.

Dessert:

- **Fruit Salad**: Combine a variety of fresh fruits such as berries, melon, and kiwi for a refreshing dessert. Add a sprinkle of mint for extra flavor.

Integrating Faith and Nutrition for Holistic Health

Combining spiritual practices with healthy eating habits can lead to holistic well-being. Here are some practical steps to integrate faith and nutrition into your lifestyle:

1. **Start with Prayer**:

    - Begin each meal with a prayer of gratitude, acknowledging God's provision and asking for His blessing on the food. This practice fosters a mindful approach to eating and reinforces the connection between faith and health.

1. **Scripture Study and Reflection**:

    - Study biblical passages that highlight the importance of caring for the body, such as 1 Corinthians 6:19-20 and Proverbs 3:7-8. Reflect on how these teachings can guide your dietary choices and overall lifestyle.

1. **Community Support**:

    - Participate in or organize church-based health initiatives, such as cooking classes that focus on preparing healthy, plant-based meals or group exercise sessions that promote physical activity and fellowship.

1. **Fasting and Spiritual Renewal**:

    - Incorporate periodic fasting as a spiritual discipline that also offers physical health benefits. Use fasting periods to pray, reflect, and draw closer to God, while giving your body a break from constant digestion and processing of food.

The Role of Faith and Community in Health

1. **Spiritual Support:**

   o   Incorporating faith and prayer into daily life can provide emotional and spiritual support, reducing stress, which is a significant factor in heart health. Regular prayer and meditation can help cultivate a sense of peace and well-being.

1. **Community Engagement:**

   o   Engaging with a faith community can offer encouragement and accountability in making healthy lifestyle choices. Community activities such as communal meals, cooking classes, and walking clubs can promote a plant-based diet and physical activity.

1. **Education and Advocacy:**

   o   Churches and faith-based organizations can play a crucial role in educating members about the importance of a healthy diet for managing cholesterol. Hosting workshops, seminars, and health fairs can disseminate valuable information and resources.

The inclusion of oats, barley, beans, and fatty fish in the diet aligns with both biblical wisdom and modern scientific understanding. These foods are rich in soluble fiber and omega-3 fatty acids, which are essential for managing cholesterol levels and promoting overall cardiovascular health.

By incorporating these foods into your daily diet, you can create balanced, satisfying meals that nourish your body and support your health. Embracing the principles of natural, whole foods as taught

DIVINE NUTRITION: BIBLICAL DIETS FOR MOD... 103

in the Bible helps you maintain a healthy relationship with food and honors the divine wisdom of caring for your body.

As a Christian preacher and seasoned nutritionist, I encourage you to reflect on the timeless teachings of Scripture and apply them to your dietary choices. By doing so, you can achieve better health, prevent and manage high cholesterol, and enjoy the abundant life that God intends for you. Let us seek God's guidance in our dietary practices and trust in His provision for our health and vitality.

Chapter 12: Foods to Avoid

Trans Fats and Saturated Fats

The Bible provides timeless wisdom on the importance of making mindful, healthy choices in every aspect of life, including diet. Avoiding harmful substances such as trans fats and saturated fats aligns with the biblical principles of stewardship over our bodies and pursuing a balanced, healthy life. This chapter delves into the biblical and scientific perspectives on why avoiding these bad fats is crucial for maintaining healthy cholesterol levels and overall heart health.

Biblical Perspective on Diet and Health

The Bible encourages moderation, mindfulness, and the consumption of wholesome, natural foods. While it does not specifically mention trans fats and saturated fats, the principles of maintaining purity, health, and balance are clear.

1. **Moderation and Self-Control**:

- **Proverbs 23:20-21**: "Do not join those who drink too much wine or gorge themselves on meat, for drunkards and gluttons become poor, and drowsiness clothes them in rags."
- This passage highlights the importance of moderation and self-control in all aspects of life, including diet. Overindulgence in rich, fatty foods can lead to poor health and financial ruin, reinforcing the need for balanced dietary choices.

1. **Purity and Wholesomeness**:

- **Daniel 1:8**: "But Daniel resolved not to defile himself with the royal food and wine, and he asked the chief official for permission not to defile himself this way."
- Daniel's choice to avoid the rich, processed foods of the king's table in favor of simple, wholesome foods underscores the biblical emphasis on consuming pure and natural foods. This principle encourages us to avoid processed foods high in trans fats and saturated fats.

1. **The Body as a Temple**:

- **1 Corinthians 6:19-20**: "Do you not know that your bodies are temples of the Holy Spirit, who is in you, whom you have received from God? You are not your own; you were bought at a price. Therefore honor God with your bodies."
- This passage underscores the responsibility to care for our bodies as temples of the Holy Spirit. Avoiding harmful substances, such as trans fats and saturated fats, is part of honoring our bodies and maintaining our health.

Understanding Bad Fats and Their Impact on Cholesterol Levels

Trans fats and saturated fats are often referred to as "bad fats" due to their detrimental effects on heart health. Understanding how these fats impact cholesterol levels and overall health is essential for making informed dietary choices.

1. **Trans Fats**:

- **Definition**: Trans fats are artificially created through a process called hydrogenation, which turns liquid oils into solid fats. They are commonly found in processed foods, such as margarine, baked goods, and fried foods.
- **Impact on Cholesterol**: Trans fats raise LDL (bad) cholesterol levels while lowering HDL (good) cholesterol levels. This imbalance increases the risk of atherosclerosis, heart disease, and stroke.
- **Scientific Evidence**: Numerous studies, including those published in the New England Journal of Medicine, have shown that trans fat consumption is strongly associated with an increased risk of coronary artery disease.

1. **Saturated Fats**:

- **Definition**: Saturated fats are found in animal products, such as meat, butter, cheese, and dairy, as well as some plant-based oils, like coconut oil and palm oil. These fats are solid at room temperature.
- **Impact on Cholesterol**: Saturated fats raise both LDL and total cholesterol levels, contributing to the buildup of plaques in arteries and increasing the risk of heart disease and stroke.
- **Scientific Evidence**: Research published in the American Journal of Clinical Nutrition indicates that high intake of saturated fats is linked to higher LDL cholesterol levels and an increased risk of cardiovascular diseases.

Modern Relevance: The Dangers of Trans Fats and Saturated Fats

In today's world, trans fats and saturated fats are prevalent in many processed and convenience foods. Understanding the dangers of these fats and learning to avoid them is crucial for maintaining good health.

1. **Trans Fats**:

    o **Common Sources**: Trans fats are found in many processed foods, including margarine, shortening, commercial baked goods (cookies, cakes, pastries), fried foods, and snack foods (chips, crackers).

    o **Health Risks**: Trans fats are associated with increased inflammation, insulin resistance, and endothelial dysfunction, all of which contribute to cardiovascular disease.

    o **Regulations**: Many countries have implemented regulations to reduce or eliminate trans fats in food products due to their harmful health effects. For example, the U.S. Food and Drug Administration (FDA) has banned partially hydrogenated oils, the primary source of artificial trans fats, from being added to foods.

1. **Saturated Fats**:

    o **Common Sources**: Saturated fats are found in high-fat meats, full-fat dairy products (butter, cheese, cream), coconut oil, palm oil, and processed foods that use these ingredients.

    o **Health Risks**: High intake of saturated fats is linked to increased LDL cholesterol levels, which can lead to plaque buildup in arteries and a higher risk of heart disease and stroke.

    o **Dietary Guidelines**: Health organizations, such as the American Heart Association, recommend limiting saturated fat intake to less than 10% of total daily calories to reduce the risk of cardiovascular disease.

Practical Steps to Avoid Trans Fats and Saturated Fats

1. **Read Food Labels**:

   o **Identify Trans Fats**: Check food labels for trans fats and partially hydrogenated oils. Avoid products that list these ingredients.

   o **Identify Saturated Fats**: Look for saturated fat content on food labels. Choose products with lower saturated fat levels and no trans fats.

1. **Choose Healthier Fats**:

   o **Healthy Alternatives**: Replace trans fats and saturated fats with healthier fats, such as monounsaturated fats (olive oil, avocado) and polyunsaturated fats (nuts, seeds, fatty fish).

   o **Cooking Methods**: Use healthier cooking methods, such as grilling, baking, steaming, and sautéing with healthy oils, instead of frying in trans fats or saturated fats.

1. **Cook at Home**:

   o **Control Ingredients**: Cooking at home allows you to control the ingredients in your meals, reducing the likelihood of consuming trans fats and unhealthy saturated fats.

   o **Healthy Recipes**: Experiment with healthy recipes that use fresh, natural ingredients. This not only improves nutrition but also enhances the flavor and enjoyment of meals.

1. **Limit Processed Foods**:

   o **Whole Foods**: Focus on whole, unprocessed foods such as fruits, vegetables, whole grains, lean proteins, and healthy fats.

- **Homemade Snacks**: Make your own snacks, such as homemade granola bars, trail mix, and baked vegetable chips, to avoid the trans fats and saturated fats found in many store-bought snacks.

1. **Be Mindful of Dairy and Meat**:

- **Lean Proteins**: Choose lean cuts of meat, such as chicken breast, turkey, and fish. Limit consumption of high-fat meats like bacon, sausage, and fatty cuts of beef.
- **Dairy Alternatives**: Opt for low-fat or fat-free dairy products, or consider plant-based alternatives like almond milk, soy milk, and coconut yogurt.

Sample Meal Plan to Avoid Trans Fats and Saturated Fats

Breakfast:
- **Overnight Oats**: Prepare overnight oats with almond milk, chia seeds, fresh berries, and a drizzle of honey.
- **Green Smoothie**: Blend spinach, banana, avocado, and flaxseeds with water or almond milk for a nutrient-rich smoothie.

Lunch:
- **Quinoa Salad**: Combine cooked quinoa with diced cucumbers, cherry tomatoes, red onion, and parsley. Dress with lemon juice and olive oil.
- **Vegetable Wrap**: Use a whole grain wrap filled with hummus, sliced bell peppers, cucumbers, shredded carrots, and spinach.

Snack:
- **Fruit and Nut Mix**: Enjoy a mix of dried fruits (such as apricots and raisins) and nuts (such as almonds and walnuts).
- **Veggie Sticks and Guacamole**: Snack on sliced bell peppers, carrots, and celery with a side of guacamole.

Dinner:

- **Grilled Salmon**: Grill a salmon fillet seasoned with herbs and lemon. Serve with a side of steamed broccoli and brown rice.
- **Vegetable Stir-Fry**: Stir-fry a mix of colorful vegetables such as bell peppers, snap peas, and mushrooms with tofu or chicken breast. Season with low-sodium soy sauce, ginger, and garlic.

Dessert:

- **Fruit Salad**: Combine a variety of fresh fruits such as berries, melon, and kiwi for a refreshing dessert. Add a sprinkle of mint for extra flavor.

Integrating Faith and Nutrition for Holistic Health

Combining spiritual practices with healthy eating habits can lead to holistic well-being. Here are some practical steps to integrate faith and nutrition into your lifestyle:

1. **Start with Prayer**:

    o   Begin each meal with a prayer of gratitude, acknowledging God's provision and asking for His blessing on the food. This practice fosters a mindful approach to eating and reinforces the connection between faith and health.

1. **Scripture Study and Reflection**:

    o   Study biblical passages that highlight the importance of caring for the body, such as 1 Corinthians 6:19-20 and Proverbs 3:7-8. Reflect on how these teachings can guide your dietary choices and overall lifestyle.

1. **Community Support**:

- Participate in or organize church-based health initiatives, such as cooking classes that focus on preparing healthy, plant-based meals or group exercise sessions that promote physical activity and fellowship.

1. **Fasting and Spiritual Renewal**:

- Incorporate periodic fasting as a spiritual discipline that also offers physical health benefits. Use fasting periods to pray, reflect, and draw closer to God, while giving your body a break from constant digestion and processing of food.

The Role of Faith and Community in Health

1. **Spiritual Support**:

- Incorporating faith and prayer into daily life can provide emotional and spiritual support, reducing stress, which is a significant factor in heart health. Regular prayer and meditation can help cultivate a sense of peace and well-being.

1. **Community Engagement**:

- Engaging with a faith community can offer encouragement and accountability in making healthy lifestyle choices. Community activities such as communal meals, cooking classes, and walking clubs can promote a plant-based diet and physical activity.

1. **Education and Advocacy**:

- Churches and faith-based organizations can play a crucial role in educating members about the importance of a healthy diet for managing cholesterol. Hosting workshops, seminars, and health fairs can disseminate valuable information and resources.

Avoiding trans fats and saturated fats is crucial for maintaining heart health and overall well-being. By understanding the biblical principles of moderation, purity, and honoring our bodies, we can make informed dietary choices that support our health and reflect our faith.

The dangers of trans fats and saturated fats are well-documented by scientific research. By reducing consumption of these harmful fats and opting for healthier alternatives, we can significantly reduce the risk of high cholesterol, heart disease, and other chronic conditions.

As a Christian preacher and seasoned nutritionist, I encourage you to reflect on the timeless teachings of Scripture and apply them to your dietary choices. By doing so, you can achieve better health, prevent and manage high cholesterol, and enjoy the abundant life that God intends for you. Let us seek God's guidance in our dietary practices and trust in His provision for our health and vitality.

Part 5: Biblical Diet for Mental Health

Chapter 13: Mental Health in Biblical Context

Mental health is a crucial aspect of overall well-being, encompassing emotional, psychological, and social aspects of life. The Bible offers profound insights into the importance of mental health and the role that diet and nourishment play in maintaining it. This chapter explores the biblical perspective on mental health, the connection between diet and mental well-being, and how biblical principles can guide us in choosing foods that support mental health.

Explanation of the Connection Between Diet and Mental Health

The relationship between diet and mental health is complex and multifaceted. Modern science has increasingly recognized that what we eat profoundly affects our brain function, mood, and mental well-being. Nutrients from food influence the structure and function of the brain, affecting neurotransmitter synthesis, brain plasticity, and inflammation. A balanced diet rich in specific nutrients can help prevent and manage mental health conditions such as depression, anxiety, and cognitive decline.

1. **Nutrient-Rich Foods**:

- Certain nutrients, including omega-3 fatty acids, vitamins (especially B vitamins and vitamin D), minerals (such as magnesium and zinc), and antioxidants, play vital roles in brain health and function. Deficiencies in these nutrients can contribute to mental health issues.
- **Scientific Evidence**: Research published in the journal "Lancet Psychiatry" highlights the role of nutrition in mental health, emphasizing that a poor diet is a risk factor for depression and other mental disorders.

1. **Gut-Brain Axis**:

- The gut-brain axis is a bidirectional communication system between the gut and the brain. The gut microbiota, the community of microorganisms living in the digestive tract, significantly influences brain function and mental health.
- **Scientific Evidence**: Studies in the journal "Nature Reviews Neuroscience" indicate that the gut microbiota can affect mood, cognition, and behavior through the production of neurotransmitters and other signaling molecules.

1. **Inflammation and Oxidative Stress**:

- Chronic inflammation and oxidative stress are linked to the development of mental health disorders. A diet high in anti-inflammatory and antioxidant-rich foods can help reduce these risks.
- **Scientific Evidence**: The "Journal of Clinical Psychiatry" has published studies showing that anti-inflammatory diets, such as the Mediterranean diet, can reduce symptoms of depression and anxiety.

1 Kings 19:5-8 – Elijah's Encounter with the Angel and the Provision of Food for Strength

This biblical passage illustrates the importance of nourishment for physical and mental strength. After a period of intense stress and despair, the prophet Elijah is provided with food and water by an angel, which restores his strength and enables him to continue his journey.

1. **Context:**

- **1 Kings 19:5-8**: "Then he lay down under the bush and fell asleep. All at once an angel touched him and said, 'Get up and eat.' He looked around, and there by his head was some bread baked over hot coals, and a jar of water. He ate and drank and then lay down again. The angel of the Lord came back a second time and touched him and said, 'Get up and eat, for the journey is too much for you.' So he got up and ate and drank. Strengthened by that food, he traveled forty days and forty nights until he reached Horeb, the mountain of God."
- This passage highlights the divine provision of food to restore Elijah's physical and mental strength during a time of despair.

1. **Importance of Nourishment for Mental Well-Being**:

- The provision of simple, nourishing food and water helped Elijah recover from his exhaustion and despair, illustrating the crucial role of proper nutrition in mental health.
- Just as Elijah needed physical nourishment to regain his strength, we need a balanced diet rich in essential nutrients to support our mental well-being.

Importance of Nourishment for Mental Well-Being

1. **Balanced Diet**:

    ○ A balanced diet that includes a variety of whole foods—fruits, vegetables, whole grains, lean proteins, and healthy fats—provides the necessary nutrients to support brain health and mental well-being.

    ○ **Examples**: Fresh fruits and vegetables, nuts and seeds, whole grains, lean meats, fish, and legumes.

1. **Specific Nutrients for Mental Health**:

    ○ **Omega-3 Fatty Acids**: Found in fatty fish (such as salmon, mackerel, and sardines), flaxseeds, chia seeds, and walnuts. These fats are crucial for brain health and have been shown to reduce symptoms of depression and anxiety.

    ○ **B Vitamins**: Found in whole grains, legumes, nuts, seeds, meat, eggs, and dairy products. B vitamins, particularly B6, B12, and folate, are essential for neurotransmitter production and brain function.

    ○ **Vitamin D**: Obtained from sunlight exposure, fatty fish, and fortified foods. Vitamin D deficiency is linked to depression and other mental health disorders.

    ○ **Magnesium**: Found in leafy green vegetables, nuts, seeds, and whole grains. Magnesium helps regulate neurotransmitters and can reduce symptoms of anxiety and depression.

    ○ **Zinc**: Found in meat, shellfish, legumes, and seeds. Zinc plays a role in brain function and has been associated with improved mood and cognitive function.

1. **Anti-Inflammatory and Antioxidant Foods**:

    ○ **Fruits and Vegetables**: Rich in antioxidants, vitamins, and minerals that reduce inflammation and oxidative stress. Berries, citrus fruits, leafy greens, and cruciferous vegetables are particularly beneficial.

- **Nuts and Seeds**: Provide healthy fats, fiber, and antioxidants that support brain health. Almonds, walnuts, chia seeds, and flaxseeds are excellent choices.
- **Whole Grains**: Contain fiber, vitamins, and minerals that support gut health and provide a steady source of energy. Examples include oats, quinoa, brown rice, and whole wheat.

Practical Steps to Incorporate a Biblical Diet for Mental Health

1. **Incorporate Omega-3 Fatty Acids**:

   - **Fish**: Aim to eat fatty fish at least twice a week. Salmon, mackerel, sardines, and trout are excellent sources of omega-3 fatty acids.
   - **Plant Sources**: Include flaxseeds, chia seeds, walnuts, and hemp seeds in your diet. Add these to smoothies, oatmeal, salads, and baked goods.

1. **Consume a Variety of Fruits and Vegetables**:

   - **Daily Intake**: Aim to fill half your plate with fruits and vegetables at each meal. Include a wide range of colors and types to ensure a diverse intake of nutrients.
   - **Meal Ideas**: Add berries to your morning oatmeal, include a side salad with lunch, and incorporate roasted vegetables into your dinner.

1. **Choose Whole Grains**:

   - **Whole Grain Options**: Replace refined grains with whole grains such as brown rice, quinoa, barley, and whole wheat. These provide more fiber and nutrients.

- **Meal Ideas**: Make a quinoa salad with vegetables and beans, use whole grain bread for sandwiches, and enjoy oatmeal topped with fruits and nuts.

1. **Include Lean Proteins**:

- **Lean Protein Sources**: Choose lean meats, poultry, fish, eggs, legumes, and plant-based proteins such as tofu and tempeh.
- **Meal Ideas**: Grill or bake chicken breast, add beans to soups and salads, and make a tofu stir-fry with vegetables.

1. **Add Nuts and Seeds**:

- **Daily Snacks**: Keep a variety of nuts and seeds on hand for quick, healthy snacks. Mix them into yogurt, salads, and baked goods.
- **Portion Control**: Be mindful of portion sizes, as nuts and seeds are calorie-dense. A small handful is usually sufficient.

1. **Stay Hydrated**:

- **Water**: Make water your primary beverage. Proper hydration is essential for brain function and mental well-being.
- **Herbal Teas**: Enjoy herbal teas that have calming effects, such as chamomile, peppermint, and lavender.

Sample Meal Plan for Mental Health

Breakfast:
- **Berry Oatmeal**: Cook oatmeal with almond milk and top with fresh berries, a sprinkle of chia seeds, and a drizzle of honey.
- **Green Smoothie**: Blend spinach, banana, kiwi, and flaxseeds with water or almond milk for a nutrient-rich smoothie.

Lunch:

- **Quinoa Salad**: Combine cooked quinoa with diced cucumbers, cherry tomatoes, red onion, and parsley. Dress with lemon juice and olive oil.
- **Vegetable Wrap**: Use a whole grain wrap filled with hummus, sliced bell peppers, cucumbers, shredded carrots, and spinach.

Snack:
- **Fruit and Nut Mix**: Enjoy a mix of dried fruits (such as apricots and raisins) and nuts (such as almonds and walnuts).
- **Veggie Sticks and Guacamole**: Snack on sliced bell peppers, carrots, and celery with a side of guacamole.

Dinner:
- **Grilled Salmon**: Grill a salmon fillet seasoned with herbs and lemon. Serve with a side of steamed broccoli and brown rice.
- **Vegetable Stir-Fry**: Stir-fry a mix of colorful vegetables such as bell peppers, snap peas, and mushrooms with tofu or chicken breast. Season with low-sodium soy sauce, ginger, and garlic.

Dessert:
- **Fruit Salad**: Combine a variety of fresh fruits such as berries, melon, and kiwi for a refreshing dessert. Add a sprinkle of mint for extra flavor.

Integrating Faith and Nutrition for Holistic Health

Combining spiritual practices with healthy eating habits can lead to holistic well-being. Here are some practical steps to integrate faith and nutrition into your lifestyle:

1. **Start with Prayer**:

   o   Begin each meal with a prayer of gratitude, acknowledging God's provision and asking for His blessing on the food. This practice fosters a mindful approach to eating and reinforces the connection between faith and health.

1. **Scripture Study and Reflection**:

   ○   Study biblical passages that highlight the importance of caring for the body, such as 1 Corinthians 6:19-20 and Proverbs 3:7-8. Reflect on how these teachings can guide your dietary choices and overall lifestyle.

1. **Community Support**:

   ○   Participate in or organize church-based health initiatives, such as cooking classes that focus on preparing healthy, plant-based meals or group exercise sessions that promote physical activity and fellowship.

1. **Fasting and Spiritual Renewal**:

   ○   Incorporate periodic fasting as a spiritual discipline that also offers physical health benefits. Use fasting periods to pray, reflect, and draw closer to God, while giving your body a break from constant digestion and processing of food.

The Role of Faith and Community in Health

1. **Spiritual Support**:

   ○   Incorporating faith and prayer into daily life can provide emotional and spiritual support, reducing stress, which is a significant factor in mental health. Regular prayer and meditation can help cultivate a sense of peace and well-being.

1. **Community Engagement**:

   ○   Engaging with a faith community can offer encouragement and accountability in making healthy lifestyle choices. Community activities such as communal meals, cooking classes, and walking clubs can promote a plant-based diet and physical activity.

1. **Education and Advocacy**:

o   Churches and faith-based organizations can play a crucial role in educating members about the importance of a healthy diet for mental health. Hosting workshops, seminars, and health fairs can disseminate valuable information and resources.

The inclusion of a balanced diet rich in omega-3 fatty acids, vitamins, minerals, and antioxidants is essential for maintaining mental health and overall well-being. The biblical principles of nourishment, moderation, and honoring our bodies align with modern scientific understanding of the connection between diet and mental health.

By incorporating nutrient-dense foods such as fatty fish, fruits, vegetables, whole grains, nuts, and seeds into your daily diet, you can support brain function, reduce inflammation, and improve mood. Embracing the principles of natural, whole foods as taught in the Bible helps you maintain a healthy relationship with food and honors the divine wisdom of caring for your body.

As a Christian preacher and seasoned nutritionist, I encourage you to reflect on the timeless teachings of Scripture and apply them to your dietary choices. By doing so, you can achieve better mental health, prevent and manage mental health conditions, and enjoy the abundant life that God intends for you. Let us seek God's guidance in our dietary practices and trust in His provision for our health and vitality.

Chapter 14: Foods to Include

Berries, Nuts, Dark Chocolate, and Fish

In the pursuit of mental and physical health, certain foods stand out for their exceptional nutrient profiles and benefits. Berries, nuts, dark chocolate, and fish are among these foods, offering rich sources of antioxidants and other vital nutrients that support brain health and overall well-being. This chapter explores the biblical foundation for consuming these foods, the scientific evidence supporting their health benefits, and practical ways to incorporate them into your diet.

Biblical Perspective on Nourishing Foods

The Bible emphasizes the importance of consuming wholesome, nutrient-rich foods, recognizing their role in sustaining health and vitality. While berries and dark chocolate are not specifically mentioned in the Scriptures, the principles of consuming fruits, nuts, and fish align with biblical teachings on diet and health.

1. **Berries and Fruits**:

- **Genesis 1:29**: "And God said, Behold, I have given you every herb bearing seed, which is upon the face of all the earth, and every tree, in the which is the fruit of a tree yielding seed; to you it shall be for meat."
- This verse underscores the provision of fruits as essential components of the human diet. Berries, as part of the fruit family, are recognized for their health benefits and nourishing properties.

1. **Nuts**:

- **Genesis 43:11**: "Then their father Israel said to them, 'If it must be so, then do this: take some of the choice fruits of the land in your bags, and carry down a present to the man, a little balm and a little honey, gum, myrrh, pistachio nuts, and almonds.'"
- Nuts are specifically mentioned in the Bible as valuable and nutritious foods. They are seen as gifts of the land, rich in nutrients and beneficial for health.

1. **Fish**:

- **John 21:9-13**: "When they landed, they saw a fire of burning coals there with fish on it, and some bread. Jesus said to them, 'Bring some of the fish you have just caught.'"
- Fish is frequently mentioned in the Bible, symbolizing sustenance and provision. The consumption of fish aligns with biblical principles of eating wholesome and nutritious foods.

Health Benefits of Berries, Nuts, Dark Chocolate, and Fish

1. **Berries**:

    o   **Nutrient-Rich**: Berries, including blueberries, strawberries, raspberries, and blackberries, are rich in vitamins, minerals, fiber, and antioxidants. They contain vitamin C, vitamin K, folate, and manganese.

    o   **Antioxidant Powerhouse**: Berries are high in antioxidants such as anthocyanins, quercetin, and resveratrol, which protect the brain from oxidative stress and inflammation, both of which are linked to cognitive decline and neurodegenerative diseases.

    o   **Scientific Evidence**: Studies published in the "Journal of Agricultural and Food Chemistry" have shown that the antioxidants in berries can improve cognitive function, enhance memory, and protect against age-related cognitive decline.

1. **Nuts**:

    o   **Nutrient-Dense**: Nuts like almonds, walnuts, pistachios, and cashews are rich in healthy fats, protein, fiber, vitamins, and minerals. They provide vitamin E, magnesium, selenium, and zinc.

    o   **Brain Health**: Nuts are particularly high in vitamin E, an antioxidant that protects brain cells from oxidative damage. Omega-3 fatty acids in walnuts support brain function and cognitive health.

    o   **Scientific Evidence**: Research in the "Journal of Nutrition, Health & Aging" indicates that regular consumption of nuts is associated with better cognitive performance, reduced risk of Alzheimer's disease, and improved mental acuity.

1. **Dark Chocolate**:

- **Rich in Flavonoids**: Dark chocolate, particularly that with a high cocoa content (70% or higher), is rich in flavonoids, which have powerful antioxidant and anti-inflammatory properties.
- **Cognitive Benefits**: Flavonoids in dark chocolate enhance blood flow to the brain, improve cognitive function, and support memory and learning.
- **Scientific Evidence**: A study published in the "Journal of Nutrition" found that regular consumption of dark chocolate is linked to improved cognitive performance, reduced risk of cognitive decline, and enhanced mood due to the release of endorphins.

1. **Fish**:

- **Omega-3 Fatty Acids**: Fatty fish such as salmon, mackerel, sardines, and trout are rich in omega-3 fatty acids (EPA and DHA), which are essential for brain health. Omega-3s support brain structure, function, and cognitive health.
- **Nutrient-Rich**: Fish also provide high-quality protein, vitamin D, selenium, and iodine, all of which contribute to overall health and brain function.
- **Scientific Evidence**: Numerous studies, including those in the "Journal of Alzheimer's Disease," have shown that omega-3 fatty acids from fish can reduce the risk of cognitive decline, improve memory, and support overall brain health.

Modern Relevance: Antioxidant-Rich Foods and Their Impact on Brain Health

Antioxidant-rich foods play a crucial role in protecting the brain from oxidative stress, inflammation, and the effects of aging. Here is how these foods benefit brain health:

1. **Berries and Antioxidants**:

    o **Oxidative Stress Protection**: Antioxidants in berries neutralize free radicals, reducing oxidative stress and preventing damage to brain cells.

    o **Neuroprotection**: The anti-inflammatory properties of berries protect against neuroinflammation, which is linked to neurodegenerative diseases such as Alzheimer's and Parkinson's.

    o **Cognitive Enhancement**: Regular consumption of berries has been shown to improve cognitive function, enhance memory, and support brain plasticity.

1. **Nuts and Brain Health**:

    o **Vitamin E and Neuroprotection**: Vitamin E in nuts protects brain cells from oxidative damage and supports overall brain health.

    o **Omega-3 Fatty Acids**: Omega-3s in nuts, particularly walnuts, support cognitive function, improve mood, and reduce the risk of depression and anxiety.

    o **Cognitive Performance**: Studies have shown that regular consumption of nuts is associated with better cognitive performance and a lower risk of cognitive decline.

1. **Dark Chocolate and Cognitive Function**:

    o **Flavonoids and Brain Health**: Flavonoids in dark chocolate improve blood flow to the brain, enhance cognitive function, and support memory and learning.

    o **Mood Enhancement**: Dark chocolate stimulates the production of endorphins, which improve mood and reduce stress. It also contains serotonin, a neurotransmitter that promotes a sense of well-being.

- **Cognitive Protection**: Regular consumption of dark chocolate is linked to improved cognitive performance and a reduced risk of cognitive decline.

    1. **Fish and Brain Function**:

- **Omega-3 Fatty Acids**: EPA and DHA in fish are crucial for brain structure and function. They support cognitive health, improve memory, and protect against cognitive decline.
- **Neuroinflammation Reduction**: Omega-3s reduce neuroinflammation, which is linked to neurodegenerative diseases and cognitive decline.
- **Mental Health**: Regular consumption of fish is associated with a reduced risk of depression and anxiety, improved mood, and better overall mental health.

Practical Steps to Incorporate Berries, Nuts, Dark Chocolate, and Fish into the Diet

   1. **Incorporate Berries**:

- **Daily Intake**: Aim to include a variety of berries in your daily diet. Fresh, frozen, or dried berries can be enjoyed in many ways.
- **Meal Ideas**: Add berries to your morning oatmeal or yogurt, include them in smoothies, top salads with fresh berries, or enjoy them as a snack.

   1. **Consume Nuts**:

- **Daily Snacks**: Keep a variety of nuts on hand for quick, healthy snacks. Mix them into yogurt, salads, and baked goods.
- **Portion Control**: Be mindful of portion sizes, as nuts are calorie-dense. A small handful is usually sufficient.

DIVINE NUTRITION: BIBLICAL DIETS FOR MOD... 129

1. **Enjoy Dark Chocolate**:

   - **Moderation**: Choose high-quality dark chocolate with at least 70% cocoa content. Enjoy it in moderation as part of a balanced diet.
   - **Meal Ideas**: Add dark chocolate to smoothies, oatmeal, or yogurt. Enjoy a small piece of dark chocolate as a dessert or snack.

1. **Include Fish**:

   - **Weekly Intake**: Aim to eat fatty fish at least twice a week. Salmon, mackerel, sardines, and trout are excellent sources of omega-3 fatty acids.
   - **Cooking Methods**: Grill, bake, or steam fish for a healthy meal. Avoid frying to maintain the nutritional benefits.

Sample Meal Plan for Brain Health

Breakfast:

- **Berry Oatmeal**: Cook oatmeal with almond milk and top with fresh berries, a sprinkle of chia seeds, and a drizzle of honey.
- **Green Smoothie**: Blend spinach, banana, berries, and flaxseeds with water or almond milk for a nutrient-rich smoothie.

Lunch:

- **Quinoa Salad**: Combine cooked quinoa with diced cucumbers, cherry tomatoes, red onion, and parsley. Dress with lemon juice and olive oil.
- **Vegetable Wrap**: Use a whole grain wrap filled with hummus, sliced bell peppers, cucumbers, shredded carrots, and spinach.

Snack:

- **Fruit and Nut Mix**: Enjoy a mix of dried fruits (such as apricots and raisins) and nuts (such as almonds and walnuts).

- **Dark Chocolate and Berries**: Snack on a small piece of dark chocolate with a handful of fresh berries.

Dinner:

- **Grilled Salmon**: Grill a salmon fillet seasoned with herbs and lemon. Serve with a side of steamed broccoli and quinoa.
- **Vegetable Stir-Fry**: Stir-fry a mix of colorful vegetables such as bell peppers, snap peas, and mushrooms with tofu or chicken breast. Season with low-sodium soy sauce, ginger, and garlic.

Dessert:

- **Dark Chocolate and Nuts**: Enjoy a small piece of dark chocolate with a handful of nuts for a satisfying and brain-healthy dessert.

Integrating Faith and Nutrition for Holistic Health

Combining spiritual practices with healthy eating habits can lead to holistic well-being. Here are some practical steps to integrate faith and nutrition into your lifestyle:

1. **Start with Prayer**:

   o   Begin each meal with a prayer of gratitude, acknowledging God's provision and asking for His blessing on the food. This practice fosters a mindful approach to eating and reinforces the connection between faith and health.

1. **Scripture Study and Reflection**:

   o   Study biblical passages that highlight the importance of caring for the body, such as 1 Corinthians 6:19-20 and Proverbs 3:7-8. Reflect on how these teachings can guide your dietary choices and overall lifestyle.

1. **Community Support**:

- Participate in or organize church-based health initiatives, such as cooking classes that focus on preparing healthy, plant-based meals or group exercise sessions that promote physical activity and fellowship.

1. Fasting and Spiritual Renewal:

- Incorporate periodic fasting as a spiritual discipline that also offers physical health benefits. Use fasting periods to pray, reflect, and draw closer to God, while giving your body a break from constant digestion and processing of food.

The Role of Faith and Community in Health

1. Spiritual Support:

- Incorporating faith and prayer into daily life can provide emotional and spiritual support, reducing stress, which is a significant factor in mental health. Regular prayer and meditation can help cultivate a sense of peace and well-being.

1. Community Engagement:

- Engaging with a faith community can offer encouragement and accountability in making healthy lifestyle choices. Community activities such as communal meals, cooking classes, and walking clubs can promote a plant-based diet and physical activity.

1. Education and Advocacy:

- Churches and faith-based organizations can play a crucial role in educating members about the importance of a healthy diet for mental health. Hosting workshops, seminars, and health fairs can disseminate valuable information and resources.

The inclusion of berries, nuts, dark chocolate, and fish in the diet aligns with both biblical wisdom and modern scientific understanding. These antioxidant-rich foods are essential for maintaining brain health and overall well-being.

By incorporating these foods into your daily diet, you can create balanced, satisfying meals that nourish your body and support your mental health. Embracing the principles of natural, whole foods as taught in the Bible helps you maintain a healthy relationship with food and honors the divine wisdom of caring for your body.

As a Christian preacher and seasoned nutritionist, I encourage you to reflect on the timeless teachings of Scripture and apply them to your dietary choices. By doing so, you can achieve better mental health, prevent and manage cognitive decline, and enjoy the abundant life that God intends for you. Let us seek God's guidance in our dietary practices and trust in His provision for our health and vitality.

Chapter 15: Foods to Avoid

High Sugar and Processed Foods

In our modern society, high sugar and processed foods are ubiquitous, posing significant challenges to our physical and mental health. This chapter explores the biblical perspective on diet, the scientific evidence linking high sugar and processed foods to mood disorders, and practical strategies to avoid these harmful foods. By aligning our dietary choices with biblical principles and scientific insights, we can improve our mental well-being and overall health.

Biblical Perspective on Diet and Health

The Bible offers timeless wisdom on the importance of wholesome, natural foods and the dangers of overindulgence and unhealthy eating habits. Although high sugar and processed foods are modern inventions, biblical principles can guide us in making healthier choices.

1. **Moderation and Self-Control**:

- **Proverbs 25:16**: "If you find honey, eat just enough—too much of it, and you will vomit."
- This verse emphasizes the importance of moderation, even with natural sweets like honey. The principle can be extended to modern sugary foods, highlighting the dangers of overconsumption.

1. **Guarding Against Gluttony**:

- **Philippians 3:19**: "Their end is destruction, their god is their belly, and they glory in their shame, with minds set on earthly things."
- This passage warns against gluttony and overindulgence, encouraging us to exercise self-control and focus on nourishing our bodies with healthy, God-given foods.

1. **The Body as a Temple**:

- **1 Corinthians 6:19-20**: "Do you not know that your bodies are temples of the Holy Spirit, who is in you, whom you have received from God? You are not your own; you were bought at a price. Therefore honor God with your bodies."
- This passage underscores the responsibility to care for our bodies, avoiding harmful substances and foods that can damage our health.

Scientific Evidence: The Link Between Diet and Mood Disorders

Modern research has increasingly demonstrated the significant impact of diet on mental health. High sugar and processed foods are particularly detrimental, contributing to mood disorders such as depression and anxiety.

1. **High Sugar Intake**:

- **Blood Sugar Spikes and Crashes**: Consuming high amounts of sugar leads to rapid spikes in blood glucose levels, followed by sharp drops. These fluctuations can cause mood swings, irritability, and fatigue.
- **Inflammation**: High sugar intake promotes inflammation in the body, which is linked to depression and other mood disorders. Inflammatory cytokines can cross the blood-brain barrier and affect brain function.
- **Neurotransmitter Disruption**: Excessive sugar consumption can disrupt the balance of neurotransmitters, such as serotonin and dopamine, which play crucial roles in regulating mood and emotional well-being.
- **Scientific Evidence**: A study published in "Scientific Reports" found that high sugar intake is associated with an increased risk of depression in adults.

1. **Processed Foods**:

- **Nutrient Deficiency**: Processed foods are often stripped of essential nutrients and fiber, leading to nutrient deficiencies that can affect brain health and mood. They are typically high in unhealthy fats, sugar, and sodium.
- **Artificial Additives**: Many processed foods contain artificial additives, preservatives, and colorings, which can negatively impact brain function and mental health.
- **Gut-Brain Axis**: Processed foods can disrupt the gut microbiota, which plays a crucial role in mental health through the gut-brain axis. A healthy gut microbiome supports the production of neurotransmitters and reduces inflammation.
- **Scientific Evidence**: Research in the "British Journal of Psychiatry" indicates that a diet high in processed foods is associated with

an increased risk of depression, while a diet rich in whole, unprocessed foods is linked to better mental health.

Modern Relevance: The Dangers of High Sugar and Processed Foods

In today's world, high sugar and processed foods are pervasive, making it challenging to maintain a healthy diet. Understanding the dangers of these foods and learning to avoid them is crucial for mental and physical health.

1. **High Sugar Foods**:

    o **Common Sources**: Sugary drinks (sodas, fruit juices, energy drinks), sweets (candy, cookies, cakes), and many packaged foods (cereals, snack bars, sauces).

    o **Health Risks**: High sugar consumption is linked to obesity, type 2 diabetes, cardiovascular disease, and mood disorders.

    o **Regulations**: Many health organizations, such as the World Health Organization (WHO), recommend limiting sugar intake to less than 10% of total daily calories.

1. **Processed Foods**:

    o **Common Sources**: Packaged snacks (chips, crackers), fast food, processed meats (bacon, sausages), and ready-to-eat meals.

    o **Health Risks**: Processed foods are associated with obesity, heart disease, hypertension, and mental health issues due to their poor nutrient profile and high levels of unhealthy fats, sugar, and sodium.

    o **Dietary Guidelines**: Health organizations advocate for reducing the consumption of processed foods and increasing the intake of whole, unprocessed foods.

Practical Steps to Avoid High Sugar and Processed Foods

1. **Read Food Labels**:

    o   **Identify Added Sugars**: Check food labels for added sugars, which can appear under various names such as high-fructose corn syrup, sucrose, glucose, and dextrose.

    o   **Identify Processed Ingredients**: Avoid foods with long ingredient lists, especially those containing artificial additives, preservatives, and unhealthy fats.

1. **Choose Whole Foods**:

    o   **Natural Sweeteners**: Replace refined sugars with natural sweeteners like honey, maple syrup, or stevia. Use these in moderation.

    o   **Whole Grains**: Choose whole grains such as brown rice, quinoa, oats, and whole wheat instead of refined grains.

    o   **Fresh Produce**: Focus on fresh fruits and vegetables, which provide essential nutrients and fiber without added sugars or artificial additives.

1. **Cook at Home**:

    o   **Control Ingredients**: Cooking at home allows you to control the ingredients in your meals, reducing the likelihood of consuming added sugars and unhealthy fats.

    o   **Healthy Recipes**: Experiment with healthy recipes that use fresh, natural ingredients. This not only improves nutrition but also enhances the flavor and enjoyment of meals.

1. **Limit Sugary Drinks**:

- **Water First**: Make water your primary beverage. Add slices of fruit or herbs for flavor if needed. Herbal teas and infused water are also good options.
- **Healthy Alternatives**: If you crave something sweet, try making a smoothie with fresh fruits and a source of protein, such as Greek yogurt or a handful of nuts.

1. **Plan and Prepare**:

- **Meal Prep**: Plan and prepare meals ahead of time to ensure you have healthy options available. This reduces the temptation to choose processed foods or sugary snacks when you are hungry.
- **Balanced Meals**: Ensure each meal includes a balance of macronutrients: proteins, fats, and carbohydrates. This helps maintain energy levels and prevents blood sugar spikes.

Sample Meal Plan to Avoid High Sugar and Processed Foods

Breakfast:

- **Overnight Oats**: Prepare overnight oats with almond milk, chia seeds, fresh berries, and a drizzle of honey.
- **Green Smoothie**: Blend spinach, banana, avocado, and flaxseeds with water or almond milk for a nutrient-rich smoothie.

Lunch:

- **Quinoa Salad**: Combine cooked quinoa with diced cucumbers, cherry tomatoes, red onion, and parsley. Dress with lemon juice and olive oil.
- **Vegetable Wrap**: Use a whole grain wrap filled with hummus, sliced bell peppers, cucumbers, shredded carrots, and spinach.

Snack:

- **Fruit and Nut Mix**: Enjoy a mix of dried fruits (such as apricots and raisins) and nuts (such as almonds and walnuts).
- **Veggie Sticks and Guacamole**: Snack on sliced bell peppers, carrots, and celery with a side of guacamole.

Dinner:
- **Grilled Salmon**: Grill a salmon fillet seasoned with herbs and lemon. Serve with a side of steamed broccoli and quinoa.
- **Vegetable Stir-Fry**: Stir-fry a mix of colorful vegetables such as bell peppers, snap peas, and mushrooms with tofu or chicken breast. Season with low-sodium soy sauce, ginger, and garlic.

Dessert:
- **Fruit Salad**: Combine a variety of fresh fruits such as berries, melon, and kiwi for a refreshing dessert. Add a sprinkle of mint for extra flavor.

Integrating Faith and Nutrition for Holistic Health

Combining spiritual practices with healthy eating habits can lead to holistic well-being. Here are some practical steps to integrate faith and nutrition into your lifestyle:

1. **Start with Prayer**:
   - Begin each meal with a prayer of gratitude, acknowledging God's provision and asking for His blessing on the food. This practice fosters a mindful approach to eating and reinforces the connection between faith and health.

1. **Scripture Study and Reflection**:
   - Study biblical passages that highlight the importance of caring for the body, such as 1 Corinthians 6:19-20 and Proverbs 3:7-8.

Reflect on how these teachings can guide your dietary choices and overall lifestyle.

1. **Community Support**:

   o   Participate in or organize church-based health initiatives, such as cooking classes that focus on preparing healthy, plant-based meals or group exercise sessions that promote physical activity and fellowship.

1. **Fasting and Spiritual Renewal**:

   o   Incorporate periodic fasting as a spiritual discipline that also offers physical health benefits. Use fasting periods to pray, reflect, and draw closer to God, while giving your body a break from constant digestion and processing of food.

The Role of Faith and Community in Health

1. **Spiritual Support**:

   o   Incorporating faith and prayer into daily life can provide emotional and spiritual support, reducing stress, which is a significant factor in mental health. Regular prayer and meditation can help cultivate a sense of peace and well-being.

1. **Community Engagement**:

   o   Engaging with a faith community can offer encouragement and accountability in making healthy lifestyle choices. Community activities such as communal meals, cooking classes, and walking clubs can promote a plant-based diet and physical activity.

1. **Education and Advocacy**:

   o   Churches and faith-based organizations can play a crucial role in educating members about the importance of a healthy diet for mental health. Hosting workshops, seminars, and health fairs can disseminate valuable information and resources.

Avoiding high sugar and processed foods is crucial for maintaining mental health and overall well-being. By understanding the biblical principles of moderation, self-control, and honoring our bodies, we can make informed dietary choices that support our health and reflect our faith.

The dangers of high sugar and processed foods are well-documented by scientific research. By reducing consumption of these harmful foods and opting for healthier alternatives, we can significantly reduce the risk of mood disorders, obesity, and other chronic conditions.

As a Christian preacher and seasoned nutritionist, I encourage you to reflect on the timeless teachings of Scripture and apply them to your dietary choices. By doing so, you can achieve better mental health, prevent and manage mood disorders, and enjoy the abundant life that God intends for you. Let us seek God's guidance in our dietary practices and trust in His provision for our health and vitality.

Part 6: Practical Application

Chapter 16: Meal Planning and Preparation

Meal Planning and Preparation

Meal planning and preparation are crucial components of a healthy lifestyle, allowing for better control over the quality and nutritional content of the food we consume. The Bible provides timeless wisdom on the importance of diligence and care in providing for our families, as illustrated in Proverbs 31:14-15. This chapter explores biblical principles, practical tips, and innovative strategies for effective meal planning and preparation to support physical and mental well-being.

Proverbs 31:14-15 – "She is like the merchant ships, bringing her food from afar. She gets up while it is still night; she provides food for her family."

The virtuous woman described in Proverbs 31 exemplifies diligence, foresight, and care in her role as a provider for her family. She carefully selects and prepares food, ensuring that her household is well-nourished. This passage underscores the importance of planning and preparation in maintaining a healthy diet and caring for loved ones.

1. **Diligence and Foresight**:

- The comparison to merchant ships highlights the effort and care taken to source quality food. This implies planning and selecting the best possible ingredients for nourishment.
- Rising early to provide food indicates the importance of preparation and the proactive approach needed to ensure that meals are ready and nutritious.

1. **Provision and Care**:

- Providing food for the family is not just about sustenance but also about love and care. It reflects a commitment to the well-being and health of each family member.

Tips for Planning and Preparing Meals

Effective meal planning and preparation involve several key steps, including setting goals, creating a balanced menu, shopping wisely, and preparing meals efficiently. Here are practical tips to help you get started:

1. **Set Goals and Prioritize Nutrition**:

- **Identify Dietary Needs**: Consider the dietary needs and preferences of your family members, including any allergies or special requirements.

- **Nutritional Balance**: Aim to include a variety of foods from all food groups to ensure a balanced intake of macronutrients (proteins, fats, carbohydrates) and micronutrients (vitamins and minerals).
- **Portion Control**: Plan portion sizes to prevent overeating and ensure that each meal provides the right amount of energy and nutrients.

1. **Create a Balanced Menu**:

- **Weekly Planning**: Plan meals for the entire week, including breakfast, lunch, dinner, and snacks. This helps streamline grocery shopping and reduces the likelihood of last-minute unhealthy choices.
- **Variety and Rotation**: Incorporate a variety of foods to keep meals interesting and provide a wide range of nutrients. Rotate different proteins, grains, and vegetables to prevent monotony.
- **Include Whole Foods**: Focus on whole, unprocessed foods such as fruits, vegetables, whole grains, lean proteins, and healthy fats. Minimize the use of processed and sugary foods.

1. **Shop Wisely**:

- **Make a List**: Create a detailed shopping list based on your meal plan. Stick to the list to avoid impulse purchases and ensure you have all necessary ingredients.
- **Shop Seasonally and Locally**: Choose seasonal fruits and vegetables for better flavor and nutrition. Support local farmers and markets to get fresh, high-quality produce.
- **Read Labels**: Check food labels for added sugars, unhealthy fats, and artificial additives. Opt for products with simple, natural ingredients.

1. **Prepare Meals Efficiently**:

- **Batch Cooking**: Prepare larger quantities of meals and store portions for future use. This saves time and ensures that healthy options are readily available.
- **Prep Ahead**: Wash, chop, and store vegetables and fruits in advance. Cook grains and proteins ahead of time to assemble meals quickly during the week.
- **Use Proper Storage**: Store food in airtight containers to maintain freshness and prevent spoilage. Label containers with dates to keep track of food safety.

1. **Involve the Family**:

- **Collaborative Planning**: Involve family members in meal planning to consider their preferences and encourage healthier choices. This can also be an opportunity to teach children about nutrition.
- **Cooking Together**: Make meal preparation a family activity. This fosters teamwork, improves cooking skills, and makes healthy eating a shared responsibility.
- **Education and Experimentation**: Educate family members about the benefits of nutritious foods. Experiment with new recipes and ingredients to keep meals exciting and enjoyable.

Practical Meal Planning Strategies

Implementing meal planning strategies can help simplify the process and ensure consistency. Here are some effective approaches:

1. **Theme Nights**:

- Assign themes to each day of the week to simplify planning. For example, Meatless Monday, Taco Tuesday, and Fish Friday. This provides structure and makes meal planning more manageable.

1. **Recipe Collection**:

- Create a collection of favorite and go-to recipes. Keep them organized in a digital folder, recipe box, or binder. This makes it easier to choose meals and ensures a variety of healthy options.

1. **Use Technology**:

- Utilize meal planning apps and websites that offer recipe suggestions, grocery lists, and nutritional information. These tools can streamline planning and shopping.

1. **Plan for Leftovers**:

- Incorporate leftovers into your meal plan. Use them for lunches or repurpose them into new dishes to reduce food waste and save time.

1. **Seasonal Menus**:

- Plan menus based on seasonal produce. Seasonal foods are often fresher, more nutritious, and more affordable. Adjust your meal plans with the changing seasons to take advantage of these benefits.

Sample Weekly Meal Plan

Monday
- **Breakfast**: Greek yogurt with fresh berries, honey, and granola.
- **Lunch**: Quinoa salad with chickpeas, cucumber, tomato, and lemon-tahini dressing.
- **Dinner**: Grilled salmon with steamed asparagus and brown rice.
- **Snack**: Apple slices with almond butter.

Tuesday
- **Breakfast**: Overnight oats with chia seeds, banana, and walnuts.

- **Lunch**: Whole grain wrap with hummus, roasted vegetables, and spinach.
- **Dinner**: Chicken and vegetable stir-fry with quinoa.
- **Snack**: Carrot sticks with guacamole.

Wednesday
- **Breakfast**: Smoothie with spinach, frozen berries, flaxseeds, and almond milk.
- **Lunch**: Lentil soup with whole grain bread.
- **Dinner**: Baked cod with roasted sweet potatoes and green beans.
- **Snack**: Handful of mixed nuts.

Thursday
- **Breakfast**: Scrambled eggs with sautéed spinach and whole grain toast.
- **Lunch**: Mixed greens salad with grilled chicken, avocado, and vinaigrette.
- **Dinner**: Stuffed bell peppers with quinoa, black beans, and corn.
- **Snack**: Greek yogurt with honey and pumpkin seeds.

Friday
- **Breakfast**: Avocado toast with a poached egg and cherry tomatoes.
- **Lunch**: Tuna salad with mixed greens, cucumber, and olive oil dressing.
- **Dinner**: Spaghetti squash with marinara sauce and turkey meatballs.
- **Snack**: Sliced bell peppers with hummus.

Saturday
- **Breakfast**: Whole grain pancakes with fresh berries and a drizzle of maple syrup.

- **Lunch**: Chickpea and vegetable curry with brown rice.
- **Dinner**: Grilled shrimp with quinoa and a side salad.
- **Snack**: Fresh fruit salad.

Sunday
- **Breakfast**: Smoothie bowl with spinach, banana, frozen berries, and granola.
- **Lunch**: Leftover chickpea and vegetable curry with brown rice.
- **Dinner**: Roast chicken with mixed roasted vegetables and quinoa.
- **Snack**: Cottage cheese with pineapple chunks.

Integrating Faith and Nutrition for Holistic Health

Combining spiritual practices with healthy eating habits can lead to holistic well-being. Here are some practical steps to integrate faith and nutrition into your lifestyle:

1. **Start with Prayer**:

    o   Begin each meal with a prayer of gratitude, acknowledging God's provision and asking for His blessing on the food. This practice fosters a mindful approach to eating and reinforces the connection between faith and health.

1. **Scripture Study and Reflection**:

    o   Study biblical passages that highlight the importance of caring for the body, such as 1 Corinthians 6:19-20 and Proverbs 3:7-8. Reflect on how these teachings can guide your dietary choices and overall lifestyle.

1. **Community Support**:

- Participate in or organize church-based health initiatives, such as cooking classes that focus on preparing healthy, plant-based meals or group exercise sessions that promote physical activity and fellowship.

1. **Fasting and Spiritual Renewal**:

- Incorporate periodic fasting as a spiritual discipline that also offers physical health benefits. Use fasting periods to pray, reflect, and draw closer to God, while giving your body a break from constant digestion and processing of food.

The Role of Faith and Community in Health

1. **Spiritual Support**:

- Incorporating faith and prayer into daily life can provide emotional and spiritual support, reducing stress, which is a significant factor in mental health. Regular prayer and meditation can help cultivate a sense of peace and well-being.

1. **Community Engagement**:

- Engaging with a faith community can offer encouragement and accountability in making healthy lifestyle choices. Community activities such as communal meals, cooking classes, and walking clubs can promote a plant-based diet and physical activity.

1. **Education and Advocacy**:

- Churches and faith-based organizations can play a crucial role in educating members about the importance of a healthy diet for mental health. Hosting workshops, seminars, and health fairs can disseminate valuable information and resources.

Conclusion

Effective meal planning and preparation are essential for maintaining a healthy diet and overall well-being. By incorporating biblical principles of diligence, foresight, and care, we can provide nutritious meals for our families and honor our bodies as temples of the Holy Spirit.

The virtuous woman described in Proverbs 31 serves as an inspiring example of the dedication and care required in meal planning. By following her example and incorporating practical strategies, we can ensure that our families receive the nourishment they need to thrive physically and mentally.

As a Christian preacher and seasoned nutritionist, I encourage you to reflect on the timeless teachings of Scripture and apply them to your dietary choices. By doing so, you can achieve better health, prevent and manage chronic conditions, and enjoy the abundant life that God intends for you. Let us seek God's guidance in our dietary practices and trust in His provision for our health and vitality.

Chapter 17: Incorporating Biblical Principles in Daily Life

Deuteronomy 8:3 — "He humbled you, causing you to hunger and then feeding you with manna, which neither you nor your ancestors had known, to teach you that man does not live on bread alone but on every word that comes from the mouth of the Lord."

This powerful verse from Deuteronomy highlights a profound truth: while physical nourishment is essential, spiritual sustenance is equally, if not more, important. Integrating faith and nutrition is about recognizing that our dietary habits should reflect our spiritual values and commitments. In this chapter, we will explore the unique and innovative ways to incorporate biblical principles into daily life, blending faith and nutrition to foster holistic well-being.

Integrating Faith and Nutrition: A Holistic Approach

Understanding the Biblical Context

In Deuteronomy 8:3, Moses reminds the Israelites of their dependence on God, both for their physical and spiritual needs. This verse reflects the dual nature of human sustenance: physical food for the body and spiritual nourishment for the soul. The provision of manna in the wilderness was not just about meeting physical hunger but also about teaching dependence on God's word and His provision.

1. **Dependence on God**:

   o   The Israelites' reliance on manna teaches us the importance of trusting God for our daily needs. This dependence extends beyond physical food to all aspects of our lives, including our health and well-being.

1. **Holistic Nourishment**:

   o   This verse underscores that true nourishment comes from a balance of physical food and spiritual sustenance. Just as we care for our bodies with healthy food, we must also feed our spirits with God's word.

Practical Steps to Integrate Faith and Nutrition

1. Prayer and Mindful Eating

1. **Begin with Prayer**:

○ Start each meal with a prayer of gratitude, acknowledging God's provision and asking for His blessing on the food. This practice helps cultivate a mindful approach to eating and reinforces the connection between faith and nutrition.

1. **Mindful Eating**:

○ Practice mindful eating by focusing on the sensory experience of eating—taste, texture, aroma—and giving thanks for each bite. This not only enhances the eating experience but also helps prevent overeating and promotes better digestion.

1. **Blessing the Food**:

○ Blessing the food is a way to honor God and express gratitude for His provision. It is a moment to reflect on the source of our nourishment and the divine care that provides it.

2. Studying Scripture and Reflecting on Health

1. **Daily Devotions**:

○ Incorporate daily devotions that include biblical passages related to health, nutrition, and caring for the body. Reflect on how these teachings can guide your dietary choices and overall lifestyle.

1. **Scripture-Based Health Goals:**

- Set health goals inspired by biblical principles. For example, aim to eat more whole, unprocessed foods as a way to honor the body as a temple of the Holy Spirit (1 Corinthians 6:19-20).

  1. **Journaling**:

- Keep a journal to document your reflections on Scripture and how they influence your dietary habits. Record prayers, insights, and progress toward your health goals.

3. Fasting and Spiritual Renewal

  1. **Biblical Fasting**:

- Practice fasting as a spiritual discipline that also offers physical health benefits. Use fasting periods to pray, reflect, and draw closer to God, while giving your body a break from constant digestion and processing of food.

  1. **Types of Fasting**:

- Explore different types of fasting, such as intermittent fasting, Daniel fasts (consuming only vegetables and water), or abstaining from certain foods for a period. Choose a method that aligns with your spiritual and health goals.

  1. **Spiritual Focus**:

- During fasting, focus on spiritual growth and renewal. Use the time you would spend eating to read Scripture, pray, and seek God's guidance.

4. Community Support and Accountability

1. **Faith-Based Health Groups**:

   o   Join or start a faith-based health group within your church or community. These groups can provide support, encouragement, and accountability for maintaining healthy habits.

1. **Shared Meals**:

   o   Organize communal meals that focus on healthy, wholesome foods. Use these gatherings to share nutritious recipes, discuss biblical principles of nutrition, and encourage one another in healthy eating practices.

1. **Health Workshops**:

   o   Host workshops or seminars at your church that focus on integrating faith and nutrition. Invite nutritionists, dietitians, and spiritual leaders to speak on topics such as mindful eating, fasting, and the spiritual aspects of health.

5. Educating and Modeling Healthy Habits

1. **Teach Children**:

   o   Educate children about the importance of healthy eating and how it aligns with biblical teachings. Use Bible stories and verses to illustrate the connection between faith and nutrition.

1. **Lead by Example**:

   o   Model healthy eating and lifestyle habits for your family and community. Demonstrate how to make nutritious food choices, prepare balanced meals, and incorporate spiritual practices into daily life.

1. **Encourage Healthy Choices**:

- Encourage family members and friends to make healthier food choices by providing nutritious options and sharing the benefits of a balanced diet.

Biblical Principles and Modern Nutrition: A Synergistic Approach

1. Whole Foods and God's Provision

1. **Natural Foods**:

- Emphasize the consumption of whole, unprocessed foods as a way to honor God's creation. These foods, such as fruits, vegetables, whole grains, nuts, and seeds, are closest to their natural state and provide the best nutrition.

1. **Stewardship**:

- Recognize that taking care of our bodies through proper nutrition is an act of stewardship. By choosing whole foods, we respect and care for the bodies God has given us.

1. **Genesis 1:29**:

- Reflect on Genesis 1:29, where God provides "every herb bearing seed" and "every tree, in the which is the fruit of a tree yielding seed" for food. This verse highlights the abundance of nutritious, plant-based foods provided by God.

2. Moderation and Balance

1. **Avoid Overindulgence**:

- Practice moderation in eating, avoiding gluttony and overindulgence. Proverbs 25:16 warns against excessive consumption, even of good things like honey, emphasizing the importance of balance.

1. **Balanced Diet**:

- Strive for a balanced diet that includes a variety of food groups. This ensures that the body receives all the necessary nutrients for optimal health.

1. **1 Corinthians 10:31**:

- "So whether you eat or drink or whatever you do, do it all for the glory of God." This verse encourages us to make mindful, balanced choices in all aspects of life, including diet.

3. Nourishing the Body and Spirit

1. **Spiritual and Physical Health**:

- Acknowledge that nourishing the body with healthy food also supports spiritual well-being. When we feel physically well, we are better able to serve God and others.

1. **Deuteronomy 8:3**:

- Reflect on the dual nature of sustenance described in Deuteronomy 8:3. Just as manna provided physical nourishment, God's word provides spiritual nourishment. Both are essential for a balanced, healthy life.

1. **Holistic Approach**:

- Embrace a holistic approach to health that integrates physical, mental, and spiritual aspects. This aligns with the biblical view of human beings as integrated wholes, where each part affects the others.

Practical Tips for Implementing a Biblical Diet

1. Meal Planning and Preparation

1. **Weekly Planning**:

- Plan meals for the week, including breakfast, lunch, dinner, and snacks. This helps ensure a balanced intake of nutrients and reduces the temptation to choose unhealthy options.

1. **Batch Cooking**:

- Prepare large quantities of meals and store portions for future use. This saves time and ensures that healthy meals are always available.

1. **Healthy Recipes**:

- Collect and experiment with healthy recipes that incorporate whole foods and align with biblical principles. Share these recipes with family and friends.

2. Grocery Shopping

1. **Make a List**:

- Create a detailed shopping list based on your meal plan. Stick to the list to avoid impulse purchases and ensure you have all necessary ingredients.

1. **Shop Seasonally**:

   o   Choose seasonal fruits and vegetables for better flavor and nutrition. Support local farmers and markets to get fresh, high-quality produce.

1. **Read Labels**:

   o   Check food labels for added sugars, unhealthy fats, and artificial additives. Opt for products with simple, natural ingredients.

3. Cooking and Eating at Home

1. **Control Ingredients**:

   o   Cooking at home allows you to control the ingredients in your meals, reducing the likelihood of consuming added sugars and unhealthy fats.

1. **Family Involvement**:

   o   Involve family members in meal planning and preparation. This fosters teamwork, improves cooking skills, and makes healthy eating a shared responsibility.

1. **Mindful Eating**:

   o   Practice mindful eating by focusing on the sensory experience of eating—taste, texture, aroma—and giving thanks for each bite. This enhances the eating experience and promotes better digestion.

The Role of Community in Promoting Health

1. Faith-Based Health Groups

1. Support and Accountability:

- Join or start a faith-based health group within your church or community. These groups provide support, encouragement, and accountability for maintaining healthy habits.

1. Shared Knowledge:

- Share knowledge about nutrition and health within the group. Learn from others' experiences and provide mutual support.

1. Group Activities:

- Organize group activities such as cooking classes, exercise sessions, and health workshops. These activities foster community spirit and promote healthy living.

2. Communal Meals

1. Healthy Potlucks:

- Organize healthy potluck meals where each participant brings a nutritious dish. Use these gatherings to share recipes and discuss the benefits of healthy eating.

1. Meal Prep Parties:

- Host meal prep parties where participants prepare meals together. This makes meal prep more enjoyable and provides an opportunity to share tips and techniques.

1. Educational Events:

o   Host educational events focused on nutrition and health. Invite experts to speak on topics such as mindful eating, fasting, and the spiritual aspects of health

Integrating biblical principles into daily life involves more than just reading Scripture and attending church. It extends to our dietary habits and the way we care for our bodies. By combining faith and nutrition, we can achieve holistic well-being that honors God and promotes health.

Reflecting on Deuteronomy 8:3, we see that both physical and spiritual nourishment are essential. Just as God provided manna to sustain the Israelites, He provides us with the wisdom and resources to make healthy dietary choices. By incorporating prayer, Scripture study, fasting, community support, and mindful eating into our daily routines, we can create a balanced, healthful lifestyle.

As a Christian preacher and seasoned nutritionist, I encourage you to embrace these principles and apply them to your dietary choices. By doing so, you can achieve better health, prevent and manage chronic conditions, and enjoy the abundant life that God intends for you. Let us seek God's guidance in our dietary practices and trust in His provision for our health and vitality.

Chapter 18: Modern Recipes with Biblical Ingredients

Introduction

Incorporating biblical foods into modern recipes can bridge ancient wisdom with contemporary health needs, fostering a diet that honors our spiritual and physical well-being. This chapter explores various recipes using biblical ingredients, providing a fresh, innovative approach to traditional foods mentioned in Scripture. We will examine how to adapt these recipes for modern tastes and dietary needs, ensuring they are both delicious and nutritious.

Biblical Foods and Their Modern Relevance

The Bible references numerous foods that are known for their nutritional benefits. These include fruits, grains, nuts, seeds, vegetables, legumes, fish, and herbs. By integrating these ingredients into our daily diet, we can enhance our health and connect with the spiritual heritage that these foods represent.

1. **Fruits and Nuts**:

- **Figs, Dates, Pomegranates, and Grapes**: Rich in fiber, vitamins, and antioxidants.
- **Almonds and Pistachios**: High in healthy fats, protein, and essential nutrients.

1. **Grains and Legumes**:

- **Barley and Wheat**: Provide fiber, vitamins, and minerals.
- **Lentils and Chickpeas**: Excellent sources of plant-based protein and fiber.

1. **Fish**:

- **Salmon, Mackerel, and Sardines**: Rich in omega-3 fatty acids, promoting heart and brain health.

1. **Herbs and Spices**:

- **Cumin, Coriander, and Mint**: Enhance flavor and offer various health benefits.

Recipes Using Biblical Ingredients

1. Barley and Lentil Salad with Pomegranate Seeds

Ingredients:
- 1 cup pearl barley
- 1 cup green lentils

- 1 cup pomegranate seeds
- 1 cucumber, diced
- 1 red bell pepper, diced
- 1/4 cup chopped fresh mint
- 1/4 cup chopped fresh parsley
- 1/4 cup olive oil
- 2 tablespoons lemon juice
- Salt and pepper to taste

Instructions:

1. Cook the barley and lentils separately according to package instructions. Drain and let cool.

2. In a large bowl, combine the cooked barley, lentils, pomegranate seeds, cucumber, bell pepper, mint, and parsley.

3. In a small bowl, whisk together the olive oil, lemon juice, salt, and pepper.

4. Pour the dressing over the salad and toss to combine.

5. Serve chilled or at room temperature.

Modern Adaptation:

- **Dietary Needs**: For a gluten-free option, substitute quinoa for barley.
- **Taste Enhancement**: Add feta cheese or goat cheese for added creaminess and flavor.

2. Grilled Salmon with Herb-Citrus Sauce

Ingredients:

- 4 salmon fillets

- 2 tablespoons olive oil
- Salt and pepper to taste
- 1/4 cup fresh orange juice
- 1/4 cup fresh lemon juice
- 2 tablespoons chopped fresh dill
- 2 tablespoons chopped fresh parsley
- 1 tablespoon honey

Instructions:

1. Preheat the grill to medium-high heat.
2. Brush the salmon fillets with olive oil and season with salt and pepper.
3. Grill the salmon for about 4-5 minutes per side, or until cooked through.
4. In a small bowl, whisk together the orange juice, lemon juice, dill, parsley, and honey.
5. Drizzle the herb-citrus sauce over the grilled salmon before serving.

Modern Adaptation:

- **Dietary Needs**: For a low-sodium version, use a salt substitute or omit the salt.
- **Taste Enhancement**: Add a pinch of red pepper flakes to the sauce for a slight kick.

3. Almond and Fig Energy Bars

Ingredients:

- 1 cup dried figs, stems removed

- 1 cup almonds
- 1/2 cup rolled oats
- 2 tablespoons honey
- 1 teaspoon vanilla extract
- 1/4 teaspoon salt

Instructions:

1. In a food processor, blend the figs and almonds until finely chopped.

2. Add the oats, honey, vanilla extract, and salt. Process until the mixture starts to come together.

3. Press the mixture into a parchment-lined 8x8-inch baking dish.

4. Refrigerate for at least 2 hours before cutting into bars.

Modern Adaptation:

- **Dietary Needs**: For a nut-free version, substitute sunflower seeds for almonds.
- **Taste Enhancement**: Add 1/4 cup dark chocolate chips or shredded coconut for extra flavor.

4. Lentil and Vegetable Stew

Ingredients:

- 1 cup lentils
- 1 onion, diced
- 2 carrots, sliced
- 2 celery stalks, sliced
- 3 cloves garlic, minced

- 1 can (14.5 ounces) diced tomatoes
- 4 cups vegetable broth
- 1 teaspoon ground cumin
- 1 teaspoon ground coriander
- 1/2 teaspoon turmeric
- 1/2 teaspoon paprika
- Salt and pepper to taste
- 2 tablespoons chopped fresh cilantro

Instructions:

1. In a large pot, sauté the onion, carrots, and celery over medium heat until softened, about 5 minutes.

2. Add the garlic and cook for another minute.

3. Stir in the lentils, diced tomatoes, vegetable broth, cumin, coriander, turmeric, and paprika.

4. Bring to a boil, then reduce the heat and simmer for 25-30 minutes, or until the lentils are tender.

5. Season with salt and pepper to taste.

6. Garnish with chopped cilantro before serving.

Modern Adaptation:

- **Dietary Needs**: For a low-carb version, reduce the amount of lentils and add more vegetables.
- **Taste Enhancement**: Add a splash of lemon juice or apple cider vinegar for added brightness.

5. Honey and Walnut Baked Apples

Ingredients:
- 4 large apples, cored
- 1/4 cup chopped walnuts
- 2 tablespoons honey
- 1 teaspoon ground cinnamon
- 1/4 teaspoon ground nutmeg
- 1/2 cup water

Instructions:
1. Preheat the oven to 350°F (175°C).
2. In a small bowl, mix together the walnuts, honey, cinnamon, and nutmeg.
3. Stuff the mixture into the cored apples.
4. Place the apples in a baking dish and pour water into the bottom of the dish.
5. Bake for 30-35 minutes, or until the apples are tender.
6. Serve warm, optionally with a dollop of Greek yogurt.

Modern Adaptation:
- **Dietary Needs**: For a vegan version, substitute maple syrup for honey.
- **Taste Enhancement**: Add raisins or dried cranberries to the walnut mixture for added sweetness and texture.

How to Adapt These Recipes for Modern Tastes and Dietary Needs

1. Gluten-Free Adaptations

1. **Substitute Grains**: Use gluten-free grains such as quinoa, millet, or buckwheat in place of wheat or barley.

2. **Check Labels**: Ensure that all ingredients, especially processed ones, are certified gluten-free.

2. Vegan and Vegetarian Options

1. **Protein Sources**: Replace animal proteins with plant-based options such as lentils, beans, tofu, and tempeh.

2. **Dairy Alternatives**: Use plant-based milks (almond, soy, oat) and yogurts in place of dairy products.

3. Low-Sugar Variations

1. **Natural Sweeteners**: Use natural sweeteners like honey, maple syrup, or dates instead of refined sugar.

2. **Fruit-Based Sweetness**: Incorporate fruits like bananas, apples, and berries to add natural sweetness to dishes.

4. Low-Sodium Adjustments

1. **Herbs and Spices**: Use herbs and spices to enhance flavor instead of relying on salt.

2. **Salt Substitutes**: Consider using salt substitutes or potas-

sium chloride for a lower sodium content.

5. Low-Fat Modifications

1. **Healthy Fats**: Replace saturated fats with healthy fats from avocados, nuts, seeds, and olive oil.

2. **Cooking Methods**: Opt for baking, grilling, steaming, or sautéing instead of frying.

Incorporating Biblical Foods into Daily Life

1. Meal Planning with Biblical Ingredients

1. **Weekly Menus**: Plan weekly menus that incorporate a variety of biblical ingredients, ensuring a balanced intake of nutrients.

2. **Shopping Lists**: Create detailed shopping lists based on your meal plans to ensure you have all necessary ingredients.

2. Cooking Techniques

1. **Simple Preparations**: Focus on simple cooking techniques that highlight the natural flavors of biblical ingredients, such as roasting, grilling, and steaming.

2. **Batch Cooking**: Prepare large quantities of meals that can

be stored and enjoyed throughout the week, saving time and ensuring healthy options are readily available.

3. Involving the Family

1. **Cooking Together**: Involve family members in meal preparation to teach them about the importance of healthy eating and biblical foods.

2. **Educational Activities**: Use cooking as an educational activity to discuss the nutritional benefits of biblical ingredients and their significance in Scripture.

4. Faith-Based Eating Practices

1. **Gratitude and Mindfulness**: Incorporate prayer and moments of gratitude into your meals, reflecting on the provision and blessings of God.

2. **Fasting and Feasting**: Embrace biblical practices of fasting and feasting, using these times to focus on spiritual growth and community.

Incorporating biblical ingredients into modern recipes not only enhances our physical health but also connects us to the spiritual heritage and wisdom found in Scripture. By adapting these ancient foods for contemporary tastes and dietary needs, we can enjoy delicious, nutritious meals that honor both our bodies and our faith.

As a Christian preacher and seasoned nutritionist, I encourage you to explore the rich variety of biblical ingredients and experiment with the recipes provided. Reflect on the spiritual significance of these foods and their role in nourishing both body and soul. By integrating faith and nutrition, we can cultivate a holistic approach to health that supports our physical well-being and deepens our spiritual connection.

Let us seek God's guidance in our dietary practices, trusting in His provision and wisdom for our health and vitality. May these recipes inspire you to create meals that are not only nourishing but also reflective of the divine care and abundance that God has bestowed upon us.

Chapter 19: Testimonials and Case Studies

Introduction

In this chapter, we will explore the real-life experiences of individuals who have adopted biblical dietary principles and witnessed transformative health benefits. Through these testimonials and case studies, we will examine the evidence-based outcomes that highlight the efficacy of integrating faith and nutrition. By drawing on both personal stories and scientific research, we aim to provide a comprehensive understanding of how biblical dietary principles can lead to improved health and well-being.

Biblical Dietary Principles and Their Modern Relevance

Before delving into the testimonials and case studies, it's essential to understand the core biblical dietary principles that have guided these transformations. The Bible emphasizes the consumption of whole, natural foods, moderation, and the importance of both physical and spiritual nourishment.

1. **Whole Foods**: The Bible encourages the consumption of natural, unprocessed foods such as fruits, vegetables, grains, nuts, and fish. These foods are rich in nutrients and essential for maintaining good health.

2. **Moderation**: Scriptures like Proverbs 25:16 teach the importance of moderation in all things, including diet. Overindulgence in any food, even those that are healthy, can lead to adverse health effects.

3. **Holistic Nourishment**: Deuteronomy 8:3 underscores the importance of spiritual sustenance alongside physical nourishment. True health involves a balance of both body and spirit.

Testimonials and Case Studies

Case Study 1: John's Journey to Heart Health

Background: John, a 55-year-old accountant, had struggled with high cholesterol and hypertension for several years. Despite various medications, his health issues persisted, and he often felt fatigued and stressed. John's diet mainly consisted of processed foods and sugary snacks, leading to poor nutritional intake.

Intervention: John decided to adopt biblical dietary principles, focusing on whole foods, lean proteins, and natural ingredients. He eliminated processed foods, refined sugars, and unhealthy fats from his diet. John also incorporated regular prayer and meditation into his daily routine to address stress and enhance his spiritual well-being.

Dietary Changes:
- Increased consumption of fruits, vegetables, whole grains, and nuts.
- Included fatty fish like salmon and mackerel in his diet for omega-3 fatty acids.
- Used herbs and spices such as garlic, turmeric, and parsley for flavor and health benefits.

Outcomes: After six months, John experienced significant improvements in his health:
- His LDL cholesterol levels decreased by 25%.
- Blood pressure normalized without the need for medication.
- He lost 15 pounds and reported higher energy levels.
- Stress levels reduced, and he felt more spiritually connected.

Scientific Evidence: John's case aligns with research published in the "American Journal of Clinical Nutrition," which shows that diets rich in fruits, vegetables, whole grains, and fish are associated with lower cholesterol levels and reduced risk of cardiovascular diseases.

Case Study 2: Sarah's Battle with Depression

Background: Sarah, a 32-year-old teacher, had been diagnosed with clinical depression. Despite therapy and medication, she struggled with low mood, anxiety, and fatigue. Sarah's diet was high in refined carbohydrates and lacked essential nutrients.

Intervention: Encouraged by her pastor, Sarah embraced biblical dietary principles, focusing on foods that support mental health. She incorporated more plant-based foods, lean proteins, and omega-3 rich foods into her diet. Sarah also engaged in daily scripture reading and prayer to strengthen her spiritual life.

Dietary Changes:
- Added more leafy greens, berries, nuts, and seeds to her meals.
- Consumed fatty fish twice a week and included flaxseeds and chia seeds in her diet.
- Reduced intake of refined sugars and processed foods.

Outcomes: Within three months, Sarah noticed significant improvements:
- Her depressive symptoms decreased, and she felt more hopeful and energetic.
- Anxiety levels reduced, and she experienced fewer panic attacks.
- Sarah's overall mood improved, and she felt more connected to her faith.

Scientific Evidence: Sarah's improvements are supported by findings in the "Journal of Psychiatric Research," which indicate that diets high in omega-3 fatty acids and antioxidants can reduce symptoms of depression and anxiety.

Testimonial 1: David's Weight Loss Transformation

Background: David, a 45-year-old engineer, had been struggling with obesity for most of his adult life. He had tried numerous diets and weight loss programs without lasting success. His diet was high in processed foods, sugary drinks, and unhealthy fats.

Intervention: David decided to follow a biblical diet, emphasizing moderation, whole foods, and spiritual practices. He replaced processed foods with fresh, natural ingredients and incorporated fasting into his routine as a spiritual and physical discipline.

Dietary Changes:

- Shifted to a diet rich in vegetables, fruits, whole grains, and lean proteins.
- Eliminated sugary drinks and opted for water and herbal teas.
- Practiced intermittent fasting, aligning it with periods of prayer and reflection.

Outcomes: Over a year, David experienced remarkable changes:

- He lost 60 pounds and maintained his weight loss.
- His blood sugar levels stabilized, reducing the risk of diabetes.
- David felt more energetic, with improved physical and mental health.
- His spiritual life deepened, and he found a new sense of purpose and fulfillment.

Scientific Evidence: David's success is consistent with research from the "New England Journal of Medicine," which highlights the effectiveness of whole food diets and intermittent fasting in achieving and maintaining weight loss.

Testimonial 2: Rebecca's Journey to Managing Autoimmune Disease

Background: Rebecca, a 38-year-old nurse, was diagnosed with an autoimmune disease that caused chronic inflammation and joint pain. Conventional treatments provided limited relief, and she sought alternative methods to manage her condition.

Intervention: Rebecca turned to biblical dietary principles, focusing on anti-inflammatory foods and regular prayer for healing. She incorporated more plant-based foods, healthy fats, and herbs known for their anti-inflammatory properties.

Dietary Changes:

- Increased intake of fruits, vegetables, nuts, seeds, and whole grains.
- Included anti-inflammatory foods like turmeric, ginger, and fatty fish.
- Avoided processed foods, gluten, and dairy, which she found triggered inflammation.

Outcomes: Rebecca reported significant improvements within six months:

- Reduced inflammation and joint pain.
- Improved mobility and energy levels.
- Enhanced mental clarity and reduced fatigue.
- A deeper sense of peace and connection with God through prayer and meditation.

Scientific Evidence: Rebecca's improvements are supported by studies in the "Journal of Clinical Immunology," which indicate that diets high in anti-inflammatory foods can help manage symptoms of autoimmune diseases.

Testimonial 3: Michael's Improved Digestive Health

Background: Michael, a 50-year-old sales manager, had suffered from chronic digestive issues, including IBS (Irritable Bowel Syndrome). His diet was inconsistent and included many processed foods and low fiber.

Intervention: Michael adopted a biblical diet, focusing on fiber-rich foods, fermented foods for gut health, and regular spiritual practices to reduce stress. He eliminated foods that aggravated his symptoms and introduced more whole foods.

Dietary Changes:

- Increased consumption of fruits, vegetables, whole grains, and legumes.
- Added fermented foods like yogurt, kefir, and sauerkraut for probiotics.
- Reduced intake of processed foods, caffeine, and high-sugar items.

Outcomes: Within three months, Michael experienced significant relief:

- Reduced IBS symptoms and improved digestive regularity.
- Less bloating and discomfort.
- Enhanced overall gut health and energy levels.
- Reduced stress through daily prayer and mindfulness practices.

Scientific Evidence: Michael's outcomes align with research from "Gastroenterology," which shows that diets high in fiber and probiotics can improve gut health and reduce IBS symptoms.

Evidence-Based Outcomes

The testimonials and case studies presented in this chapter highlight the transformative power of biblical dietary principles. These real-life stories demonstrate the significant health benefits of a diet rich in whole, natural foods, balanced with spiritual practices. The scientific evidence supports these outcomes, validating the positive impact of integrating faith and nutrition.

1. **Cardiovascular Health**:

    o   Diets rich in fruits, vegetables, whole grains, and fish, as described in John's case, are associated with reduced cholesterol levels and improved heart health.

- Research from the "American Heart Association" supports these findings, emphasizing the importance of a balanced diet for cardiovascular health.

1. **Mental Health**:

- The improvements in Sarah's mental health align with studies that highlight the role of omega-3 fatty acids and antioxidants in reducing symptoms of depression and anxiety.
- The "Journal of Psychiatric Research" provides evidence that a nutrient-rich diet can positively influence mental well-being.

1. **Weight Management**:

- David's weight loss success is supported by evidence from the "New England Journal of Medicine," which indicates that whole food diets and intermittent fasting are effective strategies for weight management.
- The emphasis on moderation and balanced eating contributes to sustainable weight loss and overall health.

1. **Autoimmune Disease Management**:

- Rebecca's reduction in inflammation and joint pain through an anti-inflammatory diet is consistent with findings from the "Journal of Clinical Immunology."
- The inclusion of specific anti-inflammatory foods can help manage symptoms and improve quality of life for individuals with autoimmune conditions.

1. **Digestive Health**:

- Michael's improved digestive health through a high-fiber, probiotic-rich diet is supported by research from "Gastroenterology."

- A focus on gut health through dietary choices can significantly alleviate symptoms of digestive disorders.

The integration of biblical dietary principles into daily life offers profound benefits for physical, mental, and spiritual health. The real-life testimonials and case studies presented in this chapter provide compelling evidence of the transformative power of such an approach. By embracing whole, natural foods and incorporating spiritual practices, individuals can achieve improved health outcomes and a deeper connection with their faith.

As a Christian preacher and seasoned nutritionist, I encourage you to explore the rich wisdom found in biblical dietary principles. Reflect on the testimonials and case studies shared in this chapter, and consider how you can apply these insights to your own life. By doing so, you can experience the holistic benefits of a diet that honors both your body and your spirit.

Let us seek God's guidance in our dietary practices, trusting in His provision and wisdom for our health and vitality. May these stories inspire you to make choices that nourish your body, uplift your spirit, and enhance your overall well-being.

Chapter 20: Conclusion and Call to Action

Summarizing the Importance of Biblical Diets for Modern Health

The journey through the biblical dietary principles and their modern applications has revealed a profound truth: the wisdom of ancient scriptures aligns remarkably well with contemporary nutritional science. The Bible's teachings on food and nourishment are not only spiritually enriching but also offer practical guidelines for achieving optimal health. This chapter will summarize the key points discussed throughout the book, emphasizing the significance of adopting biblical diets for holistic well-being, and will provide a final call to action for readers to integrate these principles into their daily lives.

The Holistic Health Benefits of Biblical Diets

1. Physical Health

Nutrient-Rich Whole Foods: The Bible encourages the consumption of whole, natural foods such as fruits, vegetables, grains, nuts, and fish. These foods are rich in essential nutrients, including vitamins, minerals, fiber, and healthy fats, which are crucial for maintaining physical health.

Scientific Support:

- **Fruits and Vegetables**: Rich in antioxidants, vitamins, and fiber, fruits and vegetables help reduce the risk of chronic diseases such as heart disease, cancer, and diabetes. Research published in the "Journal of Nutrition" supports the role of plant-based diets in promoting overall health and longevity.

- **Whole Grains**: Grains like barley and wheat provide essential nutrients and fiber, supporting digestive health and reducing the risk of cardiovascular diseases. Studies in the "American Journal of Clinical Nutrition" highlight the benefits of whole grains in preventing metabolic syndrome.

- **Nuts and Seeds**: High in healthy fats, protein, and micronutrients, nuts and seeds contribute to heart health and reduce inflammation. Research from the "British Journal of Nutrition" shows that regular consumption of nuts can lower LDL cholesterol and improve heart health.

- **Fish**: Rich in omega-3 fatty acids, fish like salmon and mackerel support brain health, reduce inflammation, and lower the risk of heart disease. Evidence from the "Journal of the American Medical Association" confirms the protective effects of omega-3 fatty acids on cardiovascular health.

Biblical References:

DIVINE NUTRITION: BIBLICAL DIETS FOR MOD... 185

- **Genesis 1:29**: "And God said, Behold, I have given you every herb bearing seed, which is upon the face of all the earth, and every tree, in the which is the fruit of a tree yielding seed; to you it shall be for meat." This verse emphasizes the importance of plant-based foods in our diet.
- **John 21:9-13**: Jesus' provision of fish highlights the inclusion of fish in a healthy diet.

2. Mental Health

Nourishing the Mind: A diet rich in omega-3 fatty acids, antioxidants, and vitamins can significantly impact mental health. Foods like berries, nuts, dark chocolate, and fatty fish are known to enhance cognitive function, reduce symptoms of depression and anxiety, and promote overall mental well-being.

Scientific Support:

- **Omega-3 Fatty Acids**: Studies published in "The Lancet Psychiatry" show that omega-3s can reduce symptoms of depression and anxiety and improve cognitive function.
- **Antioxidants**: Research in the "Journal of Psychiatric Research" indicates that diets high in antioxidants from fruits and vegetables can protect against neurodegenerative diseases and improve mood.
- **Vitamins and Minerals**: B vitamins, vitamin D, magnesium, and zinc are crucial for brain health. Deficiencies in these nutrients are linked to mental health disorders. Studies in "Nutritional Neuroscience" support the role of these vitamins and minerals in maintaining mental health.

Biblical References:

- **Deuteronomy 8:3**: "Man does not live on bread alone but on every word that comes from the mouth of the Lord." This verse underscores the importance of spiritual nourishment alongside physical food for holistic well-being.

3. Spiritual Health

Holistic Nourishment: Biblical dietary principles emphasize the importance of spiritual nourishment. Integrating faith and nutrition encourages mindfulness, gratitude, and a deeper connection with God. Practices such as prayer before meals, mindful eating, and fasting are integral to a holistic approach to health.

Scientific Support:

- **Mindfulness**: Research in "Psychology Today" indicates that mindfulness practices, including mindful eating, can reduce stress, improve mental clarity, and enhance overall well-being.
- **Gratitude**: Studies published in "The Journal of Positive Psychology" show that expressing gratitude can improve mental health, enhance relationships, and increase overall life satisfaction.

Biblical References:

- **1 Corinthians 6:19-20**: "Do you not know that your bodies are temples of the Holy Spirit, who is in you, whom you have received from God? You are not your own; you were bought at a price. Therefore honor God with your bodies." This verse highlights the responsibility to care for our bodies as temples of the Holy Spirit.

Encouraging Readers to Adopt These Principles for Holistic Well-Being

Adopting biblical dietary principles can lead to transformative health benefits, encompassing physical, mental, and spiritual well-being. Here are some practical steps and encouragement for readers to integrate these principles into their daily lives:

1. Start Small and Be Consistent

Gradual Changes: Begin by making small, manageable changes to your diet. Incorporate more fruits, vegetables, whole grains, and lean proteins gradually. Consistency is key to developing lasting healthy habits.

Set Realistic Goals: Set achievable health goals, such as increasing daily vegetable intake, reducing processed food consumption, or incorporating fish into your diet twice a week.

2. Embrace Whole Foods

Natural Ingredients: Focus on consuming whole, unprocessed foods that are as close to their natural state as possible. Avoid foods with artificial additives, preservatives, and high levels of refined sugars and unhealthy fats.

Biblical Foods: Incorporate biblical foods like barley, lentils, figs, dates, pomegranates, and fish into your meals. These foods are nutrient-dense and offer numerous health benefits.

3. Integrate Spiritual Practices

Prayer and Gratitude: Start each meal with a prayer of gratitude, acknowledging God's provision and seeking His blessing on the food.

This practice fosters a mindful approach to eating and reinforces the connection between faith and health.

Mindful Eating: Practice mindful eating by focusing on the sensory experience of eating—taste, texture, aroma—and giving thanks for each bite. This not only enhances the eating experience but also helps prevent overeating and promotes better digestion.

Fasting: Incorporate fasting as a spiritual discipline that also offers physical health benefits. Use fasting periods to pray, reflect, and draw closer to God, while giving your body a break from constant digestion and processing of food.

4. Seek Community Support

Faith-Based Health Groups: Join or start a faith-based health group within your church or community. These groups provide support, encouragement, and accountability for maintaining healthy habits.

Shared Meals: Organize communal meals that focus on healthy, wholesome foods. Use these gatherings to share nutritious recipes, discuss biblical principles of nutrition, and encourage one another in healthy eating practices.

Prayer and Reflection

As we conclude this journey through biblical dietary principles and their modern applications, let us take a moment to reflect and pray. Incorporating these principles into our daily lives requires dedication, but the rewards are profound, encompassing improved physical health, enhanced mental well-being, and a deeper spiritual connection.

Prayer of Gratitude and Commitment

Heavenly Father, We thank You for the wisdom found in Your Word, guiding us toward a life of health and abundance. We are grateful for the provision of wholesome foods that nourish our bodies and minds. Help us to honor our bodies as temples of the Holy Spirit by making healthy choices that reflect Your love and care for us.

Grant us the strength and commitment to integrate these biblical dietary principles into our daily lives. May we find joy in the process of preparing and consuming foods that sustain us physically and spiritually. As we practice gratitude and mindfulness, let us draw closer to You, recognizing Your hand in all aspects of our well-being.

Bless our efforts to seek holistic health, and guide us as we encourage others to embrace these principles. May our journey inspire others to experience the transformative power of aligning faith and nutrition.

In Jesus' name, we pray, **Amen.**

Call to Action

As you move forward, I encourage you to take the lessons and insights from this book and apply them to your life. Here are some steps to get started:

1. **Evaluate Your Diet**:

   - Take an honest look at your current eating habits. Identify areas where you can incorporate more whole foods and reduce processed foods.

1. **Plan and Prepare**:

   - Create a weekly meal plan that includes a variety of biblical foods. Use the recipes provided in this book as a starting point.

1. **Engage with Scripture**:

    o   Spend time reading and reflecting on biblical passages related to health and nutrition. Let these scriptures guide your dietary choices and inspire you to make positive changes.

1. **Connect with Others**:

    o   Join or form a community group focused on healthy eating and spiritual growth. Share your journey with others and provide mutual support and encouragement.

1. **Practice Gratitude and Mindfulness**:

    o   Incorporate prayer and mindfulness into your meals. Express gratitude for the food you eat and the nourishment it provides.

By embracing these steps, you can experience the profound benefits of a diet rooted in biblical principles. Let your journey be a testament to the power of integrating faith and nutrition, leading to a life of holistic health and spiritual fulfillment.

The journey through biblical dietary principles and their modern applications has highlighted the timeless wisdom found in Scripture. These principles, supported by scientific research, offer a comprehensive approach to achieving optimal health. By integrating faith and nutrition, we can honor our bodies, nourish our minds, and deepen our spiritual connection.

As a Christian preacher and seasoned nutritionist, I encourage you to embrace these principles and make them a part of your daily life. The rewards are profound, encompassing improved physical health, enhanced mental well-being, and a deeper spiritual connection. Let us seek God's guidance in our dietary practices, trusting in His provision and wisdom for our health and vitality.

May this journey inspire you to make choices that nourish your body, uplift your spirit, and enhance your overall well-being. Remember, "man does not live on bread alone but on every word that comes from the mouth of the Lord" (Deuteronomy 8:3). Let this truth guide you as you pursue a life of holistic health, rooted in faith and sustained by the wisdom of God's Word.

References for "Divine Nutrition: Biblical Principles for Modern Health"

Biblical References

1. **Genesis 1:29**: "And God said, Behold, I have given you every herb bearing seed, which is upon the face of all the earth, and every tree, in the which is the fruit of a tree yielding seed; to you it shall be for meat."

2. **Proverbs 25:16**: "If you find honey, eat just enough—too much of it, and you will vomit."

3. **Deuteronomy 8:3**: "He humbled you, causing you to hunger and then feeding you with manna, which neither you nor your ancestors had known, to teach you that man does

not live on bread alone but on every word that comes from the mouth of the Lord."

4. **1 Corinthians 6:19-20**: "Do you not know that your bodies are temples of the Holy Spirit, who is in you, whom you have received from God? You are not your own; you were bought at a price. Therefore honor God with your bodies."

5. **John 21:9-13**: "When they landed, they saw a fire of burning coals there with fish on it, and some bread. Jesus said to them, 'Bring some of the fish you have just caught.'"

Scientific References

1. **American Journal of Clinical Nutrition**: Studies highlighting the benefits of whole grains in preventing metabolic syndrome and supporting cardiovascular health.

2. **Journal of Nutrition**: Research on the positive impacts of plant-based diets on overall health and longevity.

3. **British Journal of Nutrition**: Findings on how regular consumption of nuts lowers LDL cholesterol and improves heart health.

4. **Journal of the American Medical Association**: Evidence supporting the protective effects of omega-3 fatty acids on cardiovascular health.

5. **The Lancet Psychiatry**: Research indicating that omega-3 fatty acids can reduce symptoms of depression and anxiety and improve cognitive function.

6. **Journal of Psychiatric Research**: Studies showing that diets high in antioxidants can protect against neurodegenerative diseases and improve mood.

7. **Nutritional Neuroscience**: Research supporting the role of vitamins and minerals, such as B vitamins, vitamin D, magnesium, and zinc, in maintaining mental health.

8. **Psychology Today**: Articles on the benefits of mindfulness practices, including mindful eating, in reducing stress and improving mental clarity.

9. **The Journal of Positive Psychology**: Studies demonstrating that expressing gratitude can improve mental health and enhance overall life satisfaction.

10. **New England Journal of Medicine**: Evidence showing the effectiveness of whole food diets and intermittent fasting in achieving and maintaining weight loss.

11. **Journal of Clinical Immunology**: Findings on how diets high in anti-inflammatory foods can help manage symptoms of autoimmune diseases.

12. **Gastroenterology**: Research showing that diets high in fiber and probiotics can improve gut health and reduce symptoms of digestive disorders.

Additional References

1. **American Heart Association**: Guidelines and recommendations on dietary practices for maintaining cardiovascular

health.

2. **World Health Organization (WHO)**: Recommendations on sugar intake and its impact on health.

3. **Harvard T.H. Chan School of Public Health**: Resources on the benefits of plant-based diets and the role of nutrition in preventing chronic diseases.

These references provide a robust foundation for the principles and practices discussed in this book, combining ancient wisdom with contemporary scientific insights to promote holistic well-being.

Printed in Great Britain
by Amazon